Play Therapy, CBT, DBT, and Behavior Modification Techniques for Emotional Regulation:
Helping Kids Heal from Trauma, Manage Anger and Anxiety, Build Confidence, and Strengthen Parent-Child Connection

Yevhenii Lozovyi

A Note from The Author

I hope this book will benefit you in your journey to increase your happiness and quality of life!

If you have not claimed your bonus exercise manuals, do not hesitate to email with a request. They will help you on your journey!

Note: *How to request additional exercise manuals*

Email *the subject line:* **The Book Title + exercises request.**

I do not spam! I only strive to provide value. For example, I only email monthly with a free Kindle book offer when Amazon allows me to schedule a promotion. Many books are in work now, and if you find the subject interesting, you will have a chance to receive the Kindle version for free. My main interests are mental and physical health, biohacking, and everything else that can increase happiness and quality of life.

Constructive criticism is always welcome! I am always looking for ways to improve the quality and accessibility of the materials. Feel free to reach out to

yevhenii@fiolapublishing.com

If you find this book helpful and could benefit others, please leave a review on Amazon. It would mean a word to me if you do so.

Best wishes,

Yevhenii

Contents

THE POWER OF PLAY IN NURTURING HEALTHY CHILD DEVELOPMENT

Play is far more than just a frivolous pastime - it is a vital nutrient for the growing mind, body, and spirit. Through play, children explore their world, express their feelings, build relationships, and cultivate resilience.

For children aged 6-11, the play takes on special significance as they navigate the rapid physical, cognitive, social, and emotional changes of middle childhood. Whether it's through rough-and-tumble games, imaginative adventures, or quiet crafts, play provides a safe arena for kids to test their expanding skills, roles, and ideas. Research confirms that regular playtime enhances brain development, creativity, problem-solving, emotional intelligence, social competence, and even physical health.

Importantly, play offers a unique window into children's inner worlds. The characters, themes, and conflicts that emerge in a child's play often reflect their unspoken experiences, needs and fears. When we join children in play with curiosity and acceptance, we gain profound insights into their perspectives while communicating deep empathy. Playful, responsive interactions are the foundation for secure attachment and mental wellness.

Unfortunately, many children today face barriers to accessing the benefits of play. Packed schedules, digital distractions, academic pressure, and a narrow view of play as unproductive conspire to limit kids' opportunities for free, imaginative engagement. For children already struggling with emotional or behavioral challenges, a lack of healthy play can further compound their difficulties. That's why I believe all caregivers need a robust toolkit of playful strategies to support their child's development.

UNDERSTANDING CBT, DBT, AND BEHAVIORAL MODIFICATION

In this book, we will explore how to integrate evidence-based techniques from cognitive-behavioral therapy (CBT), dialectical behavior therapy (DBT), and behavioral modification with the natural healing power of play. These well-researched modalities offer practical tools for helping kids and families navigate a wide range of mental health concerns.

At its core, CBT focuses on the interconnected relationship between thoughts, emotions and behaviors. Through CBT, children learn to notice and challenge distorted or unhelpful thinking patterns, practice coping skills for managing difficult feelings, and make positive changes in their behavior. Playful CBT activities can help kids externalize their worries, test out new self-talk, and build confidence through exposure and problem-solving.

DBT shares some features with CBT while also emphasizing mindfulness, distress tolerance, and interpersonal effectiveness. Through DBT games and role plays, kids can learn to tune into the present moment, validate their feelings while choosing adaptive behaviors, and assert their needs skillfully. These are crucial skills for children navigating intense emotions, conflicting demands, and tricky social situations.

Behavioral therapies focus on observable actions and their environmental triggers and consequences. Using praise, rewards, limit-setting, and redirection thoughtfully can help shape children's behavior in a positive direction. Playful behavioral interventions harness kids' natural motivation to engage them in learning and practicing new skills.

What makes these therapeutic approaches so valuable is that they are active, experiential, and results-oriented.

Rather than just talking about problems, children get to practice solving them through strategically designed play. With clear goals, stepwise progressions, and consistent feedback, kids build competence and confidence. Extensive research demonstrates the effectiveness of CBT, DBT, and behavioral techniques for improving outcomes for childhood anxiety, depression, anger, ADHD, autism, trauma and more.

The great news is that you don't need to be a trained clinician to apply these tools in your daily parenting! In the coming chapters, we'll explore concrete ways to embed therapeutic techniques into your play routines and interactions. By blending a spirit of lighthearted fun with proven strategies for supporting growth, you can enhance your child's coping skills and connection. Bit by a playful bit, you'll be planting the seeds for lifelong resilience.

THE SYNERGY OF PLAY THERAPY AND EVIDENCE-BASED TECHNIQUES

As a therapist, I have seen the most profound and lasting changes occur when I tap into the synergistic power of play therapy combined with evidence-based techniques like CBT, DBT, and behavioral modification. Play provides a magical gateway for making abstract therapeutic concepts concrete, memorable, and motivating for kids. Integrating these approaches allows us to harness the neurological, relational, and skill-building benefits of play to enhance clinical outcomes.

Imagine a child terrified of dogs after a frightening encounter. Through gradual, playful exposure using stuffed animals, stories and role plays, they can learn to face their fears safely while practicing coping strategies. Or picture a sibling conflict where each child is locked into black-and-white thinking. By playing out exaggerated skits of their clashing perspectives, they may discover the humor in their standoff and find space for flexibility.

In the realm of play, thoughts and feelings take on tangible, malleable forms that kids can manipulate directly. Behavioral patterns become a choose-your-own-adventure story where new possibilities unfold. Interpersonal scripts get rehearsed with the freedom to revise and ad-lib. Mastery and self-efficacy grow as kids experience themselves overcoming obstacles again and again in their pretend play.

Blending play therapy with CBT, DBT, and behavioral techniques also enhances the generalization of skills beyond the therapy room. The metaphors, games, and creative tools kids explore in session become a shared language they can apply in real-world situations. A coping skill rehearsed with a doll becomes easier to access when facing a playground challenge. Behavioral incentives linked to a favorite game hold more inherent motivation.

Crafting potent play therapy interventions grounded in evidence-based models is both an art and a science. It requires attunement to each child's developmental capacities, cultural context, and unique interests. What ignites one child's engagement may leave another indifferent. Flexibility and responsiveness are key, even as we anchor ourselves in empirically-supported practices. The beauty is that these techniques can be creatively tailored to any child's needs and passions.

EMPOWERING PARENTS AS AGENTS OF HEALING AND GROWTH

If you are a parent seeking support for your child's emotional or behavioral well-being, I commend you for your caring and commitment. I know firsthand how painful and overwhelming it can feel to watch your child struggle despite your best efforts. You may feel discouraged, drained, or at a loss for how to help. Please hear this: you are not alone, and there is hope.

As essential as professional treatment can be, I firmly believe that parents have the greatest power to facilitate their child's healing and growth. You are the expert on your unique child and family. You are the one who can take therapy tools and weave them into the fabric of daily life where kids need them most. With knowledge, practice, and self-compassion, you can learn to provide the therapeutic experiences your child needs to thrive.

That's why I have written this book specifically for parents of 6-11-year-olds. My goal is to demystify the elements of effective therapy and empower you with a flexible roadmap for playfully supporting your child's mental health. Whether your child is navigating a diagnosed condition, a situational stressor, or the ordinary challenges of growing up, the foundation is the same: a strong, secure relationship with an attuned caregiver.

In the following chapters, we will build that foundation together, one purposeful play strategy at a time. You'll gain insights into your child's developmental needs and how to assess their strengths and sticking points. You'll discover how to set thoughtful goals, craft creative interventions, and track progress. Through candid case examples and troubleshooting tips, I'll help you apply these tools flexibly and realistically.

Above all, I want to help you delight in your child again. To experience the joy, humor, and connection that flourish through shared play. To celebrate your child's hard-won gains and nurture their growing resilience. As you adopt a therapeutic approach to play, grounded in science and infused with soul, you'll be amazed at the transformation - not just in your child but in your whole family. So, let's dive in together, with playful curiosity as our guide!

Part 1: Understanding Your Child's Needs

CHAPTER 1: RECOGNIZING SIGNS AND SYMPTOMS OF EMOTIONAL STRUGGLES

SPOTTING RED FLAGS IN YOUR CHILD'S BEHAVIOR AND MOOD

As a parent, you know your child best. You are uniquely attuned to their typical ways of thinking, feeling, and behaving. So when something seems "off," it's important to pay attention. Just like physical illness, emotional struggles often manifest through observable symptoms. By learning to recognize the warning signs, you can intervene early and compassionately.

For children ages 6-12, some moodiness, fears, and acting out are par for the course. They are navigating huge cognitive, social, and identity shifts that can feel destabilizing at times. However, when behavioral and emotional changes are intense, persistent, and impairing daily functioning, they may signal a need for extra support.

Some key behavioral red flags to watch for:

- Increased aggression, defiance, or risk-taking
- Social withdrawal or isolation from friends/family
- Excessive clinginess, separation anxiety, or school refusal
- Changes in sleep (e.g., nightmares, trouble falling/staying asleep)
- Regressions in Development (e.g., baby talk, toileting accidents)
- Repetitive habits (e.g., hand washing, checking, arranging)
- Self-harm (e.g., head banging, hair pulling, cutting)

You may also notice worrisome emotional indicators like:

- Frequent worries, tearfulness or reassurance-seeking
- Harsh self-criticism, negative self-talk, or hopelessness
- Emotionally reactive - quick to anger/meltdown over minor things
- Flat or dulled affect, lack of interest or pleasure
- Physical complaints (e.g., headaches, stomachaches, fatigue)
- Hypervigilance, exaggerated startle response, flashbacks
- Perfectionism, rigid thinking, or the need for control

Now, most kids will display some of these behaviors occasionally. We all have tough days! But if you notice a significant change from your child's baseline or a cluster of symptoms persisting beyond a couple of weeks, it's worth seeking guidance. Consulting your pediatrician or a child therapist can help you tease apart transient stressors from more serious emotional struggles.

It's also crucial to consider the context around behavioral changes. Have there been any recent transitions, losses, conflicts, or traumatic events in your child's life? Are the challenges showing up in multiple domains - home, school, extracurriculars? Even a seemingly positive change, like a move or a new baby, can be a lot for a child to adjust to.

Recognize that your child may have difficulty verbalizing their inner experience at this stage. They may not yet have the emotional vocabulary or self-awareness to say, "I'm depressed" or "I'm anxious." Often, it's through externalizing behaviors that they communicate their distress and unmet needs. Your caring curiosity is the key to decoding these SOS signals.

If a significant emotional challenge seems likely, remind yourself that this is not a reflection of your parenting but an opportunity to support your child's growth. With your loving attunement and evidence-based tools, you can help them weather life's storms. In the next section, we'll explore more about how kids' mental health needs manifest through behavior and play.

THE MIND-BODY CONNECTION IN CHILDREN'S MENTAL HEALTH

As adults, we often think of mental health as residing solely in the mind. But for children, psychological distress frequently takes up residence in the body. Unexplained aches and pains, tummy troubles, fatigue, and other physical complaints are often the first signs that a child is struggling emotionally. That's because kids' developing brains and bodies are exquisitely attuned to their environment, for better or worse.

Research in developmental neuroscience has shed light on how adverse childhood experiences, whether overt trauma or chronic stress, can impact the nervous and immune systems, with ripple effects on learning, behavior, and health. When a child faces persistent threats, real or perceived, their brain and body adapt for survival. This can lead to an overactive stress response system that is quick to sound the alarm, flooding the body with fight-flight-freeze hormones.

Some common physiological manifestations of distress in children include:

- Headaches or stomachaches with no clear medical cause
- Chronic muscle tension, restlessness, or fidgeting
- Appetite changes - over or under-eating, hoarding food
- Fatigue, low energy, or motivation
- Frequent illness, lowered immunity, or trouble recovering
- Toileting issues - constipation, bed wetting, withholding
- Sensory sensitivities - easily overwhelmed by noise, lights, touch

Over time, a chronically activated stress response can make it difficult for children to discriminate between true threats and minor frustrations. They may react to everyday challenges with an intensity that seems out of proportion, cycling rapidly between fight (aggression), flight (avoidance), and freeze (shutting down). Emotional dysregulation makes it hard to self-soothe, problem-solve, or take in new information. Hypervigilance, or being constantly "on guard," can look like distractibility, irritability, and trouble sleeping.

For some children, the body becomes a battlefield for control when life feels unsafe or unpredictable. They may regulate their anxiety or anger through compulsive behaviors like hair pulling, skin picking, or active eating. Chronic stress also taxes the immune system, making kids more vulnerable to frequent or prolonged illnesses. Conversely, some children cope by disconnecting from their bodies and emotions, presenting as checked-out or unresponsive.

The mind-body connection also means that bolstering children's physical well-being is vital to supporting their mental health. Adequate sleep, nutrition, exercise, and downtime help restore equilibrium to the nervous system and build resilience. Playful movements like yoga, dance, and martial arts can discharge pent-up stress while teaching breathwork and body awareness. Predictable daily routines send cues of safety.

Parents need to advocate with schools and doctors when a child's physical symptoms are impacting their functioning. Seeking referrals to specialists like developmental pediatricians or occupational therapists can help identify underlying sensory processing or regulatory issues. An integrative approach that addresses both physical and emotional needs is key.

At the same time, a child's bodily symptoms, however distressing or disruptive, must be approached with sensitivity and acceptance. They are not acting out on purpose but attempting to cope the best they can. By listening to their body's signals with compassion, we can help kids feel seen, soothed, and safe. In the following chapter, we'll explore how to decipher the hidden logic of children's behavior and respond therapeutically.

EXERCISE 1: FEELINGS CHARADES

Objective:

This activity aims to help children and parents build emotional awareness and empathy by acting out and guessing different feeling states.

Materials:

- List of emotions
- Timer (optional)

Instructions:

1. Generate a list of age-appropriate emotions that includes a mix of comfortable and uncomfortable feelings, such as happy, sad, angry, scared, excited, worried, disappointed, and proud. You could write each emotion on index cards or slips of paper to put in a container.

2. Invite your child to play charades by explaining that the goal is to silently act out the emotions for others to guess, using facial expressions, body language, and gestures. Model an example of how to portray an emotion through acting.

3. Take turns drawing an emotion word and acting it out within a 1-2 minute time limit. Encourage players to really exaggerate their nonverbal expression of the feeling.

4. After each charade, the guesser reflects on what emotion they think was portrayed and why. The actor then shares what the intended emotion was and describes a time when they felt that way.

5. Continue taking turns until all the emotions have been acted out. Discuss any emotions that were ch___ to guess or portray, as well as any similar experiences family members have had with those feelings.

Tips:

- Emphasize that all feelings are valid and that it's okay to experience a wide range of emotions.
- Point out how different people may express the same emotion in slightly different ways.
- Make it a teaching opportunity to suggest coping strategies for uncomfortable emotions that come up.

EXERCISE 2: BODY MAP

Objective:

This activity aims to increase children's awareness of the physical sensations that accompany different emotions and to normalize body-based cues of feelings.

Materials:

- Outline of a human body (can be drawn on paper or use a life-size traced outline)
- Colored pencils, markers, or crayons

Instructions:

1. Provide your child with a printed outline of a human body or create a life-size version by tracing their body on a large piece of paper.

2. Ask your child to think about a time when they felt a strong emotion, such as excitement, sadness, or nervousness. Have them describe what was happening in their body when they had that feeling.

3. Invite them to use colors, symbols, or words to show where on the body map they experienced that emotion. For example, they might color the chest red to represent a pounding heart when scared or draw a knot in the stomach area for nervousness.

4. After mapping a few emotions, look at the body map together and reflect on what you notice. Are there any similarities or differences in how your child's body reacts to different feelings? Normalize any physical symptoms and share examples of your body-based emotional cues.

5. Discuss which physical sensations were comfortable or neutral and which ones felt uncomfortable. Brainstorm ways to release or soothe the uncomfortable sensations, such as taking slow belly breaths or relaxing tense muscles.

Tips:

- Offer to create your body map alongside your child to model emotional awareness.
- Use the body map to help your child notice when they are starting to feel overwhelmed and need to use a calming strategy.
- Refer back to the body map to build your child's emotional vocabulary and validate their physical experiences of emotions.

EXERCISE 3: MOOD METER CHECK-INS

Objective:

This activity builds emotional awareness and self-monitoring skills by having children regularly rate and track their feelings and states throughout the day.

Materials:

- Mood meter visual (can be numbers 1-10, smiley face scale, colors, or other age-appropriate rating systems)
- Journal, chart, or feelings app to record mood ratings

Instructions:

1. Introduce the mood meter concept to your child by explaining that you'll be checking in with them several times a day to see how they're feeling. Show them the rating scale you'll use, such as numbers from 1-10, a red-yellow-green stoplight visual, or faces ranging from sad to happy.

2. Decide together on regular times for mood check-ins, such as at breakfast, after school, and before bed. Set reminders if needed so you remember to invite your child to rate their mood.

3. At each designated check-in time, ask your child to pause and notice how they're feeling in that moment. Have them indicate their mood rating on the scale and record it on paper, in an app, or on a whiteboard.

4. After they rate their current feeling state, ask open-ended questions to understand more, such as "What's making you feel that way right now?" or "What do you need to help your mood?" Resist judging their rating or trying to fix their feelings.

5. At the end of each day or week, sit down together and look for any patterns in your child's recorded moods. Notice and praise their efforts at self-monitoring. Problem-solve ways to address any triggers you identify for low moods.

Tips:

- Model the mood meter for yourself by sharing your feeling ratings and coping strategies.
- Validate all of your child's emotions and emphasize that there are no "wrong" mood ratings.
- Keep the mood log somewhere accessible and visible as a reminder to pause and self-reflect.
- Consider adding an "I need..." box next to each mood rating scale where your child can indicate any support they need from you at that moment.

Remember, these exercises are just a starting point for building emotional awareness. Adapt them as needed to fit your child's developmental stage and your family's unique needs. The goal is to make talking about feelings a normal, shame-free part of your daily interactions over time.

CHAPTER 2: DECODING THE LANGUAGE OF PLAY AND BEHAVIOR

HOW CHILDREN COMMUNICATE THROUGH PLAY

As the famous child psychotherapist Garry Landreth wisely said, "Play is the child's language, and toys are their words." For children, play is not just frivolous fun but a vital means of exploring and expressing their inner world. Through the symbolic language of play, kids can communicate feelings, experiences, and needs that they may not have the verbal skills or emotional readiness to put into words.

When children feel safe and free to play spontaneously, without direction or judgment, they will often reveal the most salient themes and preoccupations of their lives. A child who has witnessed domestic violence may repeatedly crash toy cars or have superhero figures battle endlessly. One who feels powerless may play out fantasies of being trapped, rescued, or magically transformed. Lonely or anxious children may arrange toy animals in tight huddles or barricaded nests.

Children also use play to process and master challenging events. After a medical procedure or natural disaster, it's common to see kids reenact these scenarios over and over, with evolving outcomes. A child who a dog bit may have animal figures attack and injure each other, then tenderly perform surgery. In the world of imagination, they can rewrite the story's ending, find new solutions, and restore a sense of efficacy.

It's important to note that not all serious issues are present through obvious literal play. Metaphors and displacement are hallmarks of play language. A child who is being bullied may act out relational aggression between stuffed animals rather than directly representing peers. Abstract concepts like death, divorce, or moral dilemmas may be explored through generic symbols and themes like broken toys, darkness, and light, or superheroes vanquishing villains.

As you observe your child's play, notice patterns and tone as much as content. Is the play constricted, rigid or repetitive, or flexible and varied? Are characters predominantly nurturing, neglectful, aggressive, or reparative? Is the overall emotional tone anxious, frustrated, sad, or calm? How does your child's affect, energy, and engagement shift as they immerse in pretend?

Try to adopt a stance of open, accepting curiosity as you witness your child's play. Resist jumping to conclusions or making interpretations out loud. Children communicate in play because it feels indirect and less threatening than words. Asking probing questions or critiquing troubling themes is likely to shut down their fragile expression. Instead, aim to be a warm, attentive audience, narrating what you observe in brief, reflective statements. "The brave horse keeps searching for his friends." "Baby Bear looks scared and mad. He's yelling for help."

By honoring your child's play messages, however veiled or perplexing, you create permission for them to bring more of themselves to the relationship. You demonstrate that their inner reality, in all its darkness and light, is seen and accepted. This empathic foundation primes them to explore, in the safety of play, the issues that are most alive for them. In this way, decoding play language is less about nailing a precise interpretation and more about validating your child's subjective truth. From this place of feeling deeply gotten, they can begin to build bridges between their inner and outer worlds.

UNMET EMOTIONAL NEEDS AND BEHAVIORAL CLUES

Imagine a child who screams and throws his pencil every time he makes a small mistake on his homework, yelling "I'm so stupid! I hate this!" Or one who hides behind you and refuses to speak when addressed by a friendly acquaintance. Or another who frequently wakes and wanders into your room in the middle of the night. What are these behaviors trying to tell us?

On the surface, a child's actions may seem illogical, manipulative, or infuriating. It's easy to get locked into power struggles, applying generic rewards and consequences that fail to address their deepest drivers. But when we learn to look beneath the hood of challenging behaviors, we often discover a tangle of unmet emotional needs fueling the engine.

Every child has core needs for safety, security, autonomy, competence, and connection. When these needs are thwarted by circumstance or by gaps in skill, kids resort to problematic behaviors as smoke signals. A child who melts down over minor errors may be grasping for a sense of competence in the face of learning challenges. One who ignores social bids may be defending against the vulnerability of connection due to early attachment ruptures. The child creeping into your bed may be seeking the safety and soothing he's unable to provide for himself.

In other words, challenging behaviors serve a function, however dysfunctional they may appear. They are the child's best attempt to cope with and communicate distressing feelings like anxiety, anger, frustration, or loneliness. Misbehavior is a code that, once cracked, reveals the child's most urgent emotional needs and lacunae in ability.

The key is to respond to the need, not just the deed. When we react only to the surface behavior, with lectures or time-outs, we miss the opportunity to address its root cause. The child feels misunderstood, and their distress often amplifies, leading to an escalating cycle of acting out and punishment.

But when we pause to decode the unmet need or skill deficit behind a behavior, we unlock new avenues for supporting the child's growth. We search for ways to build their sense of competence rather than just demanding compliance. We proactively feed their hunger for our time and attention rather than doling it out conditionally. We co-regulate their big emotions through soothing play rather than trying to stamp them out.

This is not to say behaviors shouldn't have boundaries and consequences. Clear, consistent limits create a necessary sense of containment and safety, especially for kids who struggle with self-control. However, consequences in the absence of connection usually breed more resentment than reflection. By coupling firmness with curiosity about the meaning of the child's misbehavior, we accomplish that magic alchemy of love - holding their highest potential while accepting their current reality.

So the next time your child's actions baffle or trigger you, take a deep breath and wonder: What unmet need or skill deficit could be driving this behavior? What is my child trying to cope with or express? How can I creatively meet that need while shaping a more adaptive response? With your insights about how kids communicate through behavior and play, you have already begun the process of decoding their most important messages. In the next chapter, I'll equip you with a powerful tool for formulating and testing hypotheses about the functions of your child's behavior.

EXERCISE 1: PLAY THEME SCAVENGER HUNT

Objective:

The goal of this activity is to help parents identify recurring themes, characters, or scenarios in their child's play that may reflect their inner world, experiences, or unmet needs.

Materials:

- Notepad and pen or digital note-taking app
- Optional: Camera or video recorder to capture play themes

Instructions:

1. For a week, set aside time each day to observe your child during their free play sessions. Try to be as unobtrusive as possible, letting them lead their play.

2. As you watch, jot down notes about any recurring themes, characters, scenarios, or emotions you notice in your child's play. For example, do they often play out rescue scenarios, recreate school situations, or engage in aggressive play?

3. Pay attention to any patterns in the roles your child assigns to themselves or others in their play. Do they tend to play the hero, the villain, the caretaker, or the baby?

4. Notice any changes in your child's play themes over the course of the week. Do certain themes emerge more on days when they seem stressed or tired?

5. At the end of the week, review your notes and reflect on what you've observed. Write down any questions or hypotheses you have about what your child's play themes might be communicating about their experiences or needs.

6. Consider sharing your reflections with your child if they are developmentally ready. Invite them to share their perceptions of their play and what it means to them.

Tips:

- Resist the urge to jump in and direct your child's play, even if the themes are concerning to you. The goal is to understand their world, not to change it.
- Look for themes that seem to evoke strong emotions in your child, as these may hold particular significance.
- Consider cultural factors that may be shaping your child's play themes and roles.

EXERCISE 2: REFRAME THE BEHAVIOR

Objective:

This activity aims to help parents look beyond a child's challenging behaviors to understand the underlying unmet needs or emotional drives that may be fueling those behaviors.

Materials:

- List of recent challenging behaviors
- Pen and paper or digital document

Instructions:

1. Make a list of 3-5 challenging behaviors you've noticed in your child recently. Focus on specific, observable actions rather than vague labels. For example: "Hit sibling when the toy was taken away" instead of "aggression."

2. For each behavior, brainstorm at least three possible unmet needs or unexpressed emotions that could be driving that behavior. Some common underlying needs include seeking attention or connection, avoiding demands, expressing autonomy, sensory stimulation, or releasing pent-up feelings.

3. Write down those hypothesized needs next to each behavior. For instance, hitting when a toy is taken could stem from unmet needs for autonomy, justice, or security in relationships.

4. For each identified need, generate ideas for how you could proactively meet that need for your child more positively. Brainstorm alternative behaviors your child could use to express that need or emotion.

5. Pick one behavior you need set to focus on first. Practice noticing when your child exhibits that behavior and validate the suspected underlying need. Guide them to use the alternative coping strategies you identified.

Tips:

- Keep an open, curious mindset when reframing behaviors. Assume there is a valid need being communicated, even if the behavior itself is inappropriate.
- Model using "I feel" statements to express your own needs and emotions during challenging moments. This can help your child build the skill of communicating needs directly.
- Involve your child in generating ideas to meet their needs when they are calm and regulated. Collaborative problem-solving builds investment.

EXERCISE 3: PLAY NARRATOR

Objective:

This activity aims to help parents practice observing and reflecting on their child's play without judgment, interpretation, or interference in order to build attunement and understanding.

Materials:

- Comfortable place to sit and observe child's play
- Curiosity and patience

Instructions:

1. Set aside at least 15 minutes to sit near your child as they engage in free play. Position yourself close enough to observe details but not so close that your child shifts their play to interact with you.

2. As your child plays, act as a sportscaster or narrator, verbally describing their actions, facial expressions, tone of voice, and any dialogue between characters. Use simple behavioral observations and avoid asking questions, offering suggestions, or inferring meaning.

3. Match your tone of voice and pacing to your child's play style and energy level. For energetic, expansive play, your narration might be faster and more upbeat. For quieter, internal play, a soft, slower voice may fit better.

4. If your child looks to you for a response, offer simple reflections like "I see" or "You're focused on stacking those blocks" rather than praise or guidance. The goal is to communicate an attentive, nonjudgmental presence.

5. After the play session, take a moment to reflect on what you noticed. What can you learn about your child's inner world from the themes, actions, and feelings you observed? Consider sharing a brief, open-ended observation and asking your child to elaborate, such as "I noticed you rescued that doll over and over. I wonder what that was like for you?"

Tips:

- Let your child's play unfold at their pace. Embrace moments of silence and resist jumping in to direct the action.
- Use "you" statements to keep the focus on the child, rather than "I" statements that insert your thoughts.
- Notice any urges you have to correct, criticize, or control your child's play. Gently redirect yourself to observing mode.
- If your child invites you to join their play, ask if they want you to take on a role or copy their actions. Follow their lead as much as possible.

Remember, the goal of sportscasting is not to teach, entertain, or evaluate. It's an opportunity to communicate "I see you. I'm here. I accept you just as you are." With practice, this nonjudgmental stance helps children feel safe to express themselves fully.

CHAPTER 3: BECOMING A DETECTIVE OF YOUR CHILD'S BEHAVIOR

THE ABCS OF FUNCTIONAL ASSESSMENT

In the last chapter, we explored how children's problematic behaviors often serve as smoke signals for unmet emotional needs or lagging skills. But in the heat of the moment, when your child is melting down or acting out, it can be hard to see past the smoke to the fire beneath. That's where the tool of functional behavior assessment comes in handy.

Functional assessment is a systematic way of gathering clues about the patterns and purpose behind a child's challenging behaviors. By playing detective, you can uncover the predictable triggers, outcomes, and hidden "payoffs" that shape when and how the behavior occurs. With this insight, you can develop a plan to proactively meet your child's needs and teach more adaptive coping strategies.

The basic building blocks of a functional assessment are the "ABCs":

- Antecedents: The events, conditions, or stimuli that occur immediately before the behavior
- Behavior: A clear, objective description of the child's specific actions
- Consequences: The reactions, results, or outcomes that follow the behavior

To conduct an ABC analysis, choose a target behavior to focus on - one that happens frequently and interferes significantly with your child's functioning. Over the course of a week, jot down the ABCs each time the concerning behavior arises, using the template provided.

For example, let's say your 8-year-old erupts into aggressive tantrums most afternoons. Here's how one incident might be recorded:

A: Asked to pause video games and start homework. The parent leaves room to take a work call.

B: The child throws the controller and kicks the desk chair repeatedly while screaming, "I hate homework! You can't make me!"

C: The parent ends the call early, returns to the room, and sends the child to take a break in their room until calm. The child eventually completes part of the homework with the parent's assistance.

As you log repeated instances, patterns will emerge in the situations that set the stage for misbehavior and the apparent outcomes that reinforce it. You may discover that your child's defiance reliably attracts your focused attention or allows them to delay a difficult task. Perhaps meltdowns are more intense when they're tired, overstimulated, or caught off guard by a transition. Each data point will add a piece to the puzzle.

It's important to remember that the "C" in ABC doesn't have to mean an intentional discipline strategy. Any consistent consequence that follows the behavior, whether purposeful or accidental, positive or negative, can strengthen it. For instance, if tantrums frequently result in a sibling giving up a desired toy to keep the peace, that access to the prized possession is still reinforcing the outburst, even though you didn't plan it that way.

Of course, the A-B-C sequence is not always as linear or apparent as it looks on paper. Behavior is multiply determined, and a single outburst may serve many functions. The key is to notice the most salient patterns related to timing, setting, triggers and results. Subtle shifts in your child's facial expression, tone of voice, and body language can also provide valuable clues to their emotional state before, during, and after the behavior.

Armed with your ABC data, you're well on your way to formulating a hypothesis about why the behavior keeps happening and what your child is trying to communicate or accomplish. In the next section, we'll deepen this investigation into the functions or hidden motives that drive their most perplexing actions. The game is afoot!

UNCOVERING THE "WHY" BEHIND YOUR CHILD'S ACTIONS

In our scenario with the homework refusal tantrum, the ABC data suggests that something about the demand to transition from a preferred activity (video games) to a challenging task (homework), especially when parental assistance is lost, sets the stage for an outburst. The tantrum, in turn serves to delay the hated homework and regain dedicated parent attention, as the parent must cut their call short to help the child calm down. But how do we translate these correlations into an actionable hypothesis?

Behavior analysts have identified four main functions or "whys" that explain most problematic behaviors:

1. Attention: The behavior reliably attracts increased social interaction or focus from others, whether positive (concern, assistance) or negative (reprimands, arguing)

2. Escape: The behavior allows the child to avoid, delay, or end an undesired activity, situation, or sensory stimulation

3. Access to Tangibles: The behavior results in the child gaining an object, activity, or privilege they find rewarding

4. Sensory Stimulation: The behavior itself produces an internally pleasing or calming sensation, such as the feeling of rocking or hand flapping

Most behaviors serve multiple overlapping functions in different contexts. Our homework-battling child's tantrums seem to be maintained by both a desire for undivided parental attention and an urge to escape a taxing demand. The trick is to consider how these broad behavioral functions connect to your child's specific skill deficits and unmet physical or emotional needs.

Perhaps the child feels incapable of meeting academic expectations independently and is desperate to have you sit with them and break down the steps. The tantrum could be a misguided attempt to restore a sense of connection and competence. Or maybe they become overstimulated by the rapid removal of a soothing activity (video games) and the pressure of a non-preferred task. The aggression might be the only way they know to communicate: "Slow down, I'm feeling overwhelmed!"

As you ponder the functions of your child's behavior, consider these guiding questions:

- Does my child have the skills to meet this expectation without extra support?
- Is my child craving closeness and individual attention from me or others?
- Does my child understand what to do in this situation and why it matters to me?
- Is my child feeling powerless, out of control, or disconnected from their preferences?
- Could my child be over- or under-stimulated by sensory aspects of the environment?
- Has my child had opportunities to have their needs or opinions heard and respected?

The answers can point to which needs must be prioritized and proactively met to reduce problematic behaviors at the source. If a sense of competency is the hidden heart of the homework battle, preparing the child for the transition, providing frequent positive feedback, and collaboratively problem-solving challenges may ease their urge to fight. If dysregulation is at the root, strategies like scheduled breaks, redirection to calming activities, and a written plan for earning game time after homework could soothe their system.

Identifying the payoffs your child derives from misbehavior - the adult equivalents of workplace bonuses and health benefits - also reveals the adaptive alternatives you must offer instead. The behaviors you want to see more of, like requesting help calmly or taking a break before melting down, need to "compete" favorably with the perks of aggression. Providing your focused presence, escape options, incentives, and sensory aids for positive behaviors stacks the deck in their favor.

This is not to say you should cave to your child's every demand to avoid a tantrum. Firm, consistent boundaries are vital for their sense of safety and self-control. But by digging below the surface of the misbehavior to decode its meaning and the missing skills it signifies, you can respond with both limits and empathy. Your curious compassion is the secret sauce that helps your consequences and teaching sink in.

So dust off that deerstalker cap and put your ABC detective skills to work! By combining your intimate knowledge of your child's inner world with these behavioral sleuthing tools, you'll soon be an expert at reading between the lines of their most puzzling conduct. In the next chapter, we'll explore how to translate these insights into an action plan with your child's buy-in.

EXERCISE 1: ABC LOG

Objective:

The purpose of this activity is to help parents identify patterns in their child's challenging behaviors by systematically tracking the Antecedents (triggers), Behaviors, and Consequences of specific incidents.

Materials:

- ABC Log template (see example below)
- Pen or digital document

Instructions:

1. Create an ABC Log template or print out a pre-made one. The log should have columns for Date/Time, Antecedent, Behavior, and Consequence.

2. Over the course of a week, fill out the log each time your child exhibits a challenging behavior you want to understand better. Try to complete the entry as soon as possible after the incident while the details are fresh in your mind.

3. In the Antecedent column, write down what happened immediately before the behavior occurred. What was your child doing? Who else was present? Were there any changes in routine or environment? Be as specific and objective as possible.

4. In the Behavior column, describe your child's actions in clear, measurable terms. Instead of vague labels like "meltdown," write the specific behaviors you observed, such as "screamed, threw toys, kicked door."

5. In the Consequence column, note what happened immediately after the behavior. How did you or others respond? What changed in the environment as a result of the behavior?

6. After a week of tracking, analyze your log for patterns. Do certain triggers seem to precede the behavior more often? Are there similarities in how others respond after the behavior?

7. Use your insights to generate hypotheses about the function or purpose the behavior might be serving for your child. Is it a way to get attention, avoid a demand, or cope with overwhelming emotions? Identifying the patterns can guide your response.

Example ABC Log:

Date/Time	Antecedent	Behavior	Consequence
5/1 3 pm	Told to turn off the video game	Screamed "No!", threw the controller, kicked the door	Siblings yelled at them, a parent gave a reminder of the rules and had them pick up the controller
5/2 7 pm	Asked to put the plate in the dishwasher	Whined, "Why do I have to do everything?" and stomped off	Parent called them back and insisted they complete the task before playing

Tips:

- Be as objective and specific as possible in your log. Avoid making interpretations or judging the behavior.
- Look for patterns over time rather than concluding a single incident.
- Share relevant findings with other caregivers to get their input and ensure consistency in response.

EXERCISE 2: "WHAT'S MY FUNCTION?" GAME

Objective:

This game playfully introduces the concept of behavior functions to children and gets them thinking about the reasons behind people's actions.

Materials:

- Index cards
- Pen
- Whiteboard or paper to keep score (optional)

Instructions:

1. Before playing, brainstorm a list of behaviors you commonly see in children, such as hitting, yelling, sharing toys, hugging, etc. Write each behavior on an index card.

2. Introduce the game to your child by explaining that all behaviors have a purpose or reason behind them. Share that the four main reasons people do things are to get attention, get something they want, avoid something they don't like, or cope with uncomfortable feelings.

3. Hold up one of the behavior cards and ask your child to guess what the purpose of that behavior might be. Have them pick from the four functions: attention, tangible, escape, or coping.

4. If your child guesses correctly, offer enthusiastic feedback and a point if you're keeping score. If they guess incorrectly, validate their idea and offer a brief explanation of the most likely function.

5. Take turns drawing behavior cards and guessing functions. Offer bonus points for creative or insightful explanations of why a behavior might serve that function.

6. After the game, debrief with your child about what they noticed. Point out how the same behavior could have different purposes depending on the context. Ask them to reflect on the reasons behind some of their behaviors.

Example behaviors and functions:

- Hitting: attention, tangible, coping
- Yelling: attention, escape, coping
- Sharing: attention, tangible
- Hugging: attention, coping

Tips:

- Adapt the language and examples to your child's developmental level.
- Avoid labeling behaviors as "good" or "bad." Frame them as meeting a valid need in an unhelpful way.
- Acknowledge that behaviors can serve multiple functions and may not fit neatly into one category.

EXERCISE 3: HYPOTHESIS MAKER

Objective:

This activity helps parents practice generating and testing hypotheses about the functions of their child's behaviors in order to respond more effectively.

Materials:

- Completed ABC logs
- Hypothesis Maker template (see example below)
- Pen or digital document

Instructions:

1. Review your ABC logs and select a specific challenging behavior to focus on. Create a Hypothesis Maker template with columns for Behavior, Possible Functions, Evidence For, Evidence Against, and Experiment.

2. In the Behavior column, clearly describe the challenging behavior you want to understand better.

3. In the Possible Functions column, brainstorm at least three theories for why your child might be engaging in this behavior. Consider the four main functions: attention, tangible, escape, or coping.

4. For each hypothesis, fill in the Evidence For and Evidence Against columns with data from your ABC logs or observations. What patterns or contextual factors support or refute that particular function?

5. Based on your evidence, select the hypothesis that seems most likely. In the Experiment column, devise a plan to test this theory. How can you safely modify the triggers or consequences to see if the behavior changes in the expected direction?

6. Implement your experiment and observe the results. If your hypothesis was correct, brainstorm replacement behaviors or coping strategies to address that need more appropriately. If the behavior doesn't change as predicted, consider testing your next most likely hypothesis.

Example Hypothesis Maker:

Behavior	Possible Functions	Evidence For	Evidence Against	Experiment
Escape from non-preferred task	Behavior stops when demand is removed	Sometimes persists after the task is done		Offer a choice of 2 fun activities to do after clean up. Observe if behavior decreases.
Attention from parent	The behavior continues even when ignored	This can occur when alone in a room		

Tips:

- Be patient and persistent. It may take multiple rounds of hypothesis testing to land on the right function.
- Collaborate with other caregivers to ensure consistent data collection and experimental planning.
- Celebrate successes and learn from failed hypotheses. Both outcomes bring you closer to understanding your child.

Remember, becoming a behavior detective takes practice and flexibility. By modeling curiosity and data-driven problem solving, you teach your child invaluable skills for making sense of their own and others' behaviors. Enjoy the process of uncovering clues and cracking the case together!

CHAPTER 4: COLLABORATING WITH YOUR CHILD TO SET GOALS

DEFINING REALISTIC EXPECTATIONS AND MEASURABLE OBJECTIVES

Now that you've donned your detective cap and cracked some of the codes behind your child's behavior, you may be eager to leap into action. But before we get carried away with visions of a tantrum-free future, let's pause to get clear on exactly where we're headed and why. Just as a cross-country road trip is smoother with a well-marked map, your child's behavior change journey will be less bumpy if guided by specific, achievable goals.

When it comes to managing challenging behaviors, it's tempting to set lofty, ambitious expectations. Fueled by frustration (and perhaps a few too many parenting blogs), you may aspire for your child to go from daily explosive outbursts to Zen-master levels of calm overnight. But much like crash diets and "get rich quick" schemes, these overly optimistic goals often fizzle out fast, leaving everyone demoralized.

The key to sustainable behavior change is to aim for progress, not perfection. This means breaking down broad, long-term wishes into bite-sized, observable goals that can be realistically achieved in a short time frame. Rather than vaguely vowing to "manage anger better," zero in on a specific coping strategy you want to see more of, like "take three deep breaths when feeling frustrated before reacting."

Measurable goals allow you to objectively track your child's improvement and celebrate each small success along the way. Instead of moving the goalpost, you can high-five each other every time they manage to walk away instead of lashing out, even if it's just once a week at first. These mini-milestones build momentum and confidence, paving the way for bigger leaps.

To craft realistic, measurable goals, try using this simple formula:

"My child will exhibit X behavior under Y conditions, Z times per day/week/month."

For instance:

"My child will use 'I feel' statements to express emotions, with prompting during daily check-ins, at least 3 times this week."

"My child will independently choose a calming activity from their 'chill-out menu' when overwhelmed, before having a meltdown, 2 times per day."

Notice these goals focus more on the positive behaviors you want to encourage rather than just the problems you want to eliminate. While reducing misbehavior is the ultimate aim, framing objectives in terms of replacement skills keeps the process hopeful and actionable.

As you define these target behaviors, consider your child's unique developmental stage, temperament, and learning style. A goal that's too abstract, advanced, or out of sync with their natural wiring will only breed frustration. If your child has lagging skills in multiple domains, resist the urge to tackle them all at once. Please choose one or two high-impact priorities so you can devote your full energy to teachable moments when they arise.

This is also where your insights from the previous chapter about behavioral functions come in handy. Suppose you've hypothesized that your child's tantrums serve to escape overwhelming demands and garner your focused attention. In that case, your goals might center around distress tolerance strategies and positive ways to request support. If sensory overstimulation seems to be a trigger, you might target self-regulation skills and environmental accommodations. Always consider the need beneath the behavior you want to shift.

Of course, setting effective goals is not a solo endeavor. Your child is the main character in this adventure, and their buy-in is essential for behavior change to stick. In the next section, we'll explore how to engage your child as an active collaborator in the goal-setting process. Together, you'll map out a shared vision for a happier, more harmonious family life that you can work towards one purposeful step at a time.

ENGAGING YOUR CHILD'S COOPERATION AND MOTIVATION

If you're parenting a strong-willed 6 to 12-year-old, the idea of calmly collaborating on behavior goals may seem about as plausible as herding cats. Your child may be more interested in arguing about screen time limits than discussing strategies for emotional regulation. However, as challenging as it can be to engage a schoolager in reflection, their participation is a key predictor of success. After all, it's their behavior - and their brain - that you're aiming to shape.

One way to invite your child into the goal-setting process is to use playful, age-appropriate prompts that tap into their imagination and natural desire for autonomy. The Miracle Question, a classic technique from Solution-Focused Brief Therapy, is a great place to start:

"Imagine that while you're sleeping tonight, a magical wizard comes and waves his wand, making all the problems that brought us here disappear. When you wake up tomorrow morning, what will be the first small sign that the wizard has visited? What will be different in our family?"

This whimsical frame encourages kids to envision their ideal outcomes without getting bogged down in past failures or perceived obstacles. By describing observable changes, like "I'll get ready for school without yelling" or "I'll tell jokes at dinner instead of picking on my sister," they essentially write their own goals. You can then build on their ideas with specific action steps and incentives.

Another child-friendly way to gauge motivation and track progress is the scaling question. Using a simple 1-10 scale (where 1 is "not at all" and 10 is "completely"), ask your child to rate their current status and desired level for a target behavior:

"On a scale of 1 to 10, where 1 means 'I'm not handling frustration at all' and 10 means 'I'm a master at staying calm,' where would you say you are now with managing frustration? Where would you like to be in a week? What would that look like?"

Having your child physically plot their ratings on a colorful chart or "feelings thermometer" makes the abstract concrete. It also highlights movement towards goals, even if it's not a straight line. If they slide backward from a 6 to a 4, you can wonder aloud about what helped them climb higher before and how to recapture those conditions.

No matter how you invite your child's input, the key is to integrate their voice in a way that promotes ownership and agency. Validate their perspective ("I know it's really hard to calm down once you're super upset") while holding hope for new possibilities ("I wonder if there's a way to notice frustration early before it becomes a tornado"). Brainstorm experiment ideas together, emphasizing that there are no wrong answers and you're figuring it out as a team.

As you craft goals collaboratively, look for ways to harness your child's natural interests as incentives. If they love Minecraft, could they earn extra virtual building time to practice coping strategies? If they're obsessed with dinosaurs, could you gamify their progress on a reward chart with stickers of their favorite species? The more you can align target behaviors with your child's internal motivations, the less you'll have to rely on bribes or threats.

Remember, the goal-setting process is not a one-time event but an ongoing conversation. As your child's skills and challenges evolve, so too will their objectives and action plans. Regularly check in with your budding collaborator to celebrate wins, troubleshoot slips, and adjust course as needed. By modeling curiosity and flexibility in the face of setbacks, you'll teach them that growth is a journey, not a destination.

With your detective toolkit fully stocked and your goals firmly in sight, you're ready to embark on the heart of this book - the playful, practical interventions that will bring your aspirations to life. In the next section, we'll explore how to harness the power of therapeutic play to help your child build the skills, confidence, and connection they need to thrive. Behavior change is hard work, but with creativity, compassion, and a healthy dose of humor, it can also be full of joy. Let the games begin!

EXERCISE 1: MIRACLE QUESTION

Objective:

This activity helps children envision a future where their current problems are solved and identify concrete changes they would like to see in their lives.

Materials:

- Comfortable seating
- Optional: Drawing materials or props to enhance the miracle scenario

Instructions:

1. Invite your child to join you in a cozy spot where you can both relax and imagine together. Set a positive, hopeful tone for the activity.

2. Ask your child to close their eyes if they feel comfortable and imagine a miracle that happened overnight while they were sleeping. This miracle magically solved all of their current problems, but because they were asleep, they didn't know the miracle occurred.

3. Have your child vividly imagine waking up the morning after the miracle. Ask them to describe in detail what they would notice that's different. How would they feel in their body? What would they be doing differently? How would others respond to them?

4. Encourage your child to elaborate on the miracle scenario with specific, observable changes. Help them focus on the presence of positive activities and interactions rather than just the absence of problems.

5. After exploring the miracle, ask your child to rate on a scale of 1-10 how close they currently feel to that ideal scenario (1 being furthest away, 10 being already there). Have them describe what's already working and identify the next small steps to move up the scale.

6. Use your child's miracle responses to collaboratively set 2-3 specific, achievable goals to work towards. Write these down and post them somewhere visible as a reminder.

Tips:

- Adjust the language and scope of the miracle to your child's developmental level. Younger children may imagine a more immediate, concrete miracle, while older kids can envision longer-term changes.
- Validate any positive changes your child imagines, even if they seem small. The goal is to help them experience hope and self-efficacy.
- If your child gets stuck, offer a menu of options for changes they could make rather than leading the imagery. Allow space for their insights to emerge.

EXERCISE 2: GOAL LADDER

Objective:

This activity helps children break down big goals into manageable steps and track their progress visually to maintain motivation.

Materials:

- Paper
- Pens or markers
- Stickers or other decorations

Instructions:

1. Have your child identify a meaningful goal they want to work towards. This could be a skill they want to learn, a habit they want to develop, or a personal quality they want to embody.

2. On a piece of paper, draw a large ladder with 5-10 rungs, depending on the complexity of the goal. Write the goal at the top of the ladder.

3. Ask your child to brainstorm the specific actions or milestones needed to reach their goal, starting with the easiest step at the bottom rung and progressing to more challenging steps.

4. Help your child word each step in positive, specific terms as something they will do rather than something they will stop doing. For example, "Speak kindly to my sister" instead of "Stop calling names."

5. Have your child decorate the ladder and steps with colors, stickers, or drawings that represent their goal and motivate them to climb.

6. As your child completes each step, celebrate the accomplishment and have them color in or place a sticker on

that rung. Please encourage them to problem-solve obstacles and focus on their progress rather than the result.

7. When your child reaches the top of the ladder, affirm their success and effort. Reflect on the skills and strategies they used to overcome challenges. Have them set a new, meaningful goal to keep the momentum going.

Tips:

- Offer guidance as needed in breaking down steps, but let your child take the lead in naming them. This builds ownership and intrinsic motivation.
- Display the goal ladder somewhere prominent as a visual reminder of progress and commitment. Take a photo to share with friends and family as accountability.
- If your child loses motivation, normalize the dip and help them reconnect to their why. Focus on the next right step rather than the gap.

EXERCISE 3: FAMILY GOAL POSTER

Objective:

This collaborative activity helps families identify and visualize shared values, dreams, and intentions to foster a sense of meaning and teamwork.

Materials:

- Large poster board or butcher paper
- Magazines, printed photos, personal mementos
- Markers, paints, or other art supplies
- Glue or tape

Instructions:

1. Gather the family and explain the purpose of the activity: to create a family vision board representing your collective hopes, goals, and values.

2. Brainstorm together the key areas of life you want to represent, such as relationships, personal growth, health, spirituality, service, leisure, etc. Write these as headings around the poster.

3. Have each family member collect images, words, and objects that symbolize their individual goals and values in each area. Encourage creativity and self-expression in the representations.

4. Come together to share each person's contributions. Take turns explaining the significance of the words and pictures each member chose. Listen attentively and validate each other's aspirations.

5. Collaborate to arrange and glue the items on the poster as a unified collage. Negotiate how to represent both individual and family goals in a balanced way.

6. Once the poster is complete, display it in a central location as a daily reminder of your shared vision. Refer to it in family meetings and celebrations to affirm your progress and ongoing commitment.

7. Update the poster annually or as goals shift to maintain relevance and engagement. Notice how the family's

vision evolves as you grow together.

Tips:

- Focus on process over product. The conversations and connections that emerge during the activity are more valuable than the aesthetic of the final poster.
- Affirm each member's goals and help them frame aspirations positively. Gently challenge any representations that seem driven by avoidance or fear.
- If family members have divergent goals, look for themes of shared values that underlie them. Emphasize the unique roles each member plays in the larger family vision.

EXERCISE 4: GOAL CHARADES

Objective:

This playful activity builds perspective-taking and supports goal achievement by having family members act out and guess each other's goals.

Materials:

- Slips of paper
- Pens or pencils
- Bowl or container
- Timer (optional)

Instructions:

1. Have each family member write down 2-3 personal goals they're working towards on separate slips of paper. Fold the papers and place them in a bowl.

2. Explain the rules of charades: one person selects a goal slip from the bowl and acts it out without using words while the others guess the goal. The actor can nod or shake their head to indicate if guesses are correct.

3. Set a time limit (e.g., 2 minutes) for each round to keep the game moving. Have the goal writer keep track of the time and number of guesses.

4. Take turns drawing goal slips and acting them out. Encourage creativity and silliness in the portrayals to keep the energy light and engaging.

5. After each goal is guessed (or time runs out), have the goal writer share a bit more about why the goal is meaningful to them and what specific actions they're taking to achieve it.

6. Family members can offer encouragement, affirmation, or ideas to support the goal writer's efforts. Brainstorm how to playfully remind each other of the goals throughout the week.

7. Keep score by tracking the number of guesses per goal if desired. Celebrate the winner and all participants' vulnerability and commitment at the end.

8. Optionally, extend the activity by having members reenact each other's goals with an emphasis on the positive emotions of goal achievement. Sharing this vicarious experience can boost motivation.

Tips:

- Adapt the game for non-verbal members by using drawings, gestures, or other creative expressions.
- For young children with simpler goals, pre-write the goal ideas and have them select one to act out. Focus on goals relevant to their daily lives.
- Ensure an atmosphere of playfulness and acceptance. Redirect any teasing or criticism that may arise during guessing. The goal is to build understanding and support.

Remember, collaborative goal-setting is an ongoing process, not a one-time event. Regularly check in on goal progress during family meetings or casual conversations. Model sharing your hopes, setbacks, and successes to normalize the journey. Celebrate effort and learning as much as achievement. By making goal work playful and interpersonal, you help your child develop intrinsic motivation, grit, and a growth mindset to carry them through life's challenges.

Part 2: Therapeutic Play Techniques

CHAPTER 5: EMBRACING CHILD-CENTERED PLAY THERAPY

THE POWER OF FOLLOWING YOUR CHILD'S LEAD

Imagine for a moment that you're a child again, bursting with big feelings and even bigger dreams. In a world where grown-ups make most of the rules and plans, playtime is your sacred space to explore, experiment, and express yourself freely. It's where you go to make sense of life's joys and sorrows, to test out new roles and possibilities, and to just be wholly, unapologetically you.

As parents, we often feel the urge to guide, teach, or entertain our children during play. We suggest characters for pretend games, demonstrate the "right" way to build a tower or pepper them with questions about their artistic creations. While well-intentioned, these directing behaviors can inadvertently squelch a child's natural creativity and problem-solving. They subtly convey the message that the child's ideas are not valid or valuable unless vetted by an adult.

Child-centered play therapy (CCPT) takes a radically different approach. Developed by Virginia Axline and pioneered by luminaries like Garry Landreth, CCPT is grounded in the belief that children have an innate drive toward growth, mastery, and self-actualization. When given freedom within healthy boundaries, kids will instinctively use play to explore and express their deepest needs, desires, and strengths.

The core tenets of CCPT that distinguish it from typical play include:

1. Unconditional positive regard: Accepting and delighting in the child's unique being without judgment, evaluation, or pressure to change

2. Empathic understanding: Sensitively attuning to and reflecting the child's emotional experience and frame of reference in play

3. Child-led agenda: Trusting and following the child's lead in play, with minimal direction beyond safety limits

4. Here-and-now focus: Attending fully to the present moment of play and resisting interpretation or probing about outside events

5. Safe, consistent boundaries: Providing clear, firm limits to keep play physically and emotionally safe and predictable

In practice, this means creating a dedicated playtime (ideally at least 30 minutes a few times per week) where your child is "in charge." They decide what toys to engage with, which themes to explore, and how long to spend on each activity. Your role is to be a warm, attentive, accepting presence - to delight in their discoveries, empathize with their struggles, and trust in their journey.

Rather than praising, instructing, or asking leading questions ("What's the doggy's name? What's he building?"), your primary tool is reflective responding. This involves verbally mirroring your child's play behaviors, feelings, and desires in brief, present-tense statements:

"You're making the dinosaur stomp really hard!"

"The baby keeps getting lost. She feels scared and alone."

"You want to knock down the whole block tower, even though I'm worried it might hit me."

These empathic reflections communicate that you see, hear, and accept your child's inner world. They demonstrate that all feelings - positive and negative - are valid and manageable. Paradoxically, when kids feel free to release anger, fear, and sadness symbolically through play, the intensity of these emotions often dissipates. They shift organically to more joyful, masterful themes as their sense of safety and self-worth deepens.

Following the child's lead also means relinquishing expectations about the "right" way to use toys or create stories. A cardboard box might become a race car one minute and a robot helmet the next. Figures may have disjointed conversations or spend the whole time hiding under the couch. This fluid, non-linear play process can feel foreign to our goal-oriented adult minds. But for children, it's a vital way to experiment with power, grapple with conflicts, self-soothe, and self-organize at their own pace.

As you practice CCPT, you may marvel at the wisdom and resiliency that emerge when you trust your child's inborn creativity. You may feel tensions melt and closeness blossom as you join them in their world, just as they are. By granting them this priceless gift of unconditional acceptance, you become both their safest refuge and their launchpad to new possibilities.

But what about when play verges into unsafe territory? In the next section, we'll explore how to hold boundaries therapeutically so your child's freedom doesn't devolve into chaos or harm. With the right balance of firmness and empathy, limits can become anchors of security from which healthy exploration can thrive.

THERAPEUTIC LIMIT-SETTING AND CHOICES

One of the most common concerns parents voice about child-led play is "Won't my house get destroyed? What if they want to do something dangerous or inappropriate?" It's a valid fear - an excess of freedom without boundaries can quickly turn playtime from nourishing to nerve-racking for all involved.

But in CCPT, limits are not an afterthought or a necessary evil. They are a vital ingredient for creating the safe, predictable emotional container in which self-directed play can flourish. When kids feel confident that their exploratory urges won't catapult them into actual peril, they can surrender more fully to symbolic mastery and creative flow.

The key is to set limits proactively, minimally, and neutrally. Before playtime begins, clearly state a few essential rules that apply to every session. These should be the minimum needed to ensure physical and emotional safety for your child, yourself, and your play space.

For example:

"We need to keep each other safe. That means no hitting, throwing toys at people, or leaving this room."

"The toys in this box are for playtime. You can choose any of them and play with them however you'd like in lots of ways. If you want to play with something else, please ask first."

"When our playtime is over, I'll let you know. Then it will be time to clean up and put the toys back in the box together."

Notice these boundaries focus on observable behaviors, not on policing feelings or dictating the content of play. Your child is free to express anger, act out wild fantasies, or upend social norms - as long as it remains within the agreed-upon safety rules. Swords can clash ferociously as long as they don't touch bodies. Baby dolls can have an epic food fight as long as the play food doesn't leave the room.

When your child does approach or cross a limit, therapeutic limit-setting involves:

1. Acknowledging the feeling or wish behind the off-limits behavior
2. Firmly and kindly restating the boundary
3. Redirecting to an acceptable alternative that still honors their intent

For example:

Child: *advancing towards you aggressively with a toy sword.* "I'm gonna chop your head off!"

Parent: "You're feeling so mad, you want to attack me with that sword. I can't let you hit me; that's not safe. You can swing the sword hard at the pillows or the bear instead."

Child: *opening the door to bolt out of the playroom.* "I want to go jump on your bed!"

Parent: "You've got a lot of energy and really want to jump right now. We need to stay in this room during playtime. You could jump high like a kangaroo or make the gorilla figure jump on the toy bed in here."

This three-step process communicates empathy for the child's desires while holding reality. It grants them agency in how they express their feelings within reasonable safety constraints. If they continue to test the limit, calmly repeat the rule and redirection until they choose an acceptable path forward.

Promoting choice is another hallmark of therapeutic limit-setting. Even when options are limited, providing controlled choices gives kids a greater sense of ownership and self-determination in play. It reduces defiance by granting them some power without overwhelming them with decision fatigue.

For instance:

"It looks like you're getting tired of that game, and your body is getting wiggly. Would you like to switch to playing with the race cars or the sand tray?"

"We have five minutes left before playtime is over. Do you want me to give you a 2-minute warning or just let you know when time is up?"

By offering either/or options proactively, you help your child learn to regulate their impulses and transitions more independently. You empower them to practice self-awareness and decision-making rather than relying on you to dictate their every move.

As with all new skills, expect that your child will need lots of patient practice to internalize these limits and choices. They may repeatedly push boundaries to prove that you'll hold steady or make a mess of things because they're not used to so much autonomy. Trust that through your consistent modeling of respect, firmness, and flexibility, they are slowly building a sense of inner security and self-control.

In the playroom and life, perhaps the greatest limit we must set as parents is our urge to control, judge, and mold our children. Child-centered play invites us to embrace radical acceptance and faith in our child's unique growth journey. As we delight in their self-discovery - mud pies, imaginary perils and all - we permit them to welcome all of themselves, too. And that may be the most healing magic of all.

EXERCISE 1: SPECIAL PLAY TIME

Objective:

This activity provides a dedicated space for nondirective, child-led play that fosters autonomy, self-expression, and secure attachment.

Materials:

- Quiet, private space
- Variety of open-ended toys (e.g., blocks, figures, art supplies)
- Timer

Instructions:

1. Set aside 30-45 minutes of uninterrupted one-on-one time with your child. Explain that this is their Special Play Time, where they get to choose the activities, and you will follow their lead.

2. Provide a selection of open-ended toys that encourage imagination and creativity. Avoid toys with batteries, rules, or predetermined outcomes.

3. Allow your child to choose what and how to play. Please resist the urge to direct, teach, or correct their play. Your role is to observe, narrate, and join in as invited.

4. Follow your child's lead by imitating their actions, tone, and words. Mirror their facial expressions and energy levels to convey attunement and acceptance.

5. Reflect on your child's play using simple, descriptive statements like "You're building a tall tower" or "The bear looks sad." Avoid asking questions, making judgments, or offering interpretations.

6. Set minimal boundaries as needed to maintain physical and emotional safety. Use brief, clear statements like "I can't let you hit" or "The walls aren't for drawing on." Redirect the play gently.

7. End the session on time, even if your child protests. This maintains predictability and trust. Summarize a few key things you noticed and express excitement for your next playtime.

Tips:

- If your child invites you to play a specific role, ask for clarification on what that character would do or say. Embody the essence while letting your child control the details.
- Expect your child to test limits or express challenging emotions during play. This is a sign of safety and trust. Remain calm, consistent, and empathic in your responses.
- Keep your reflections brief and paced to avoid over-talking. Allow silences for your child to process and initiate. Trust that they will lead the way.

EXERCISE 2: PLAY THEME DECODER

Objective:

This activity helps parents identify and explore recurring themes and metaphors in their child's play as clues to their inner world and experiences.

Materials:

- Nonjudgmental curiosity
- Notebook or voice recorder (optional)
- Child's play area and toys

Instructions:

1. Observe your child's self-directed play for patterns that occur across time and activities. Notice repeating characters, scenarios, conflicts, or resolutions.

2. Consider how these play themes might symbolically represent your child's lived experiences, developmental tasks, or unmet needs. Look for parallels to recent changes, stressors, or dynamics in their world.

3. Hypothesize the "hidden messages" your child's play might be expressing about their views of self, others, and the world. What are they practicing or processing through metaphor?

4. Resist jumping to conclusions or pathologizing your child's play. Many dark or aggressive play themes are normal ways of mastering anxiety or powerlessness. Note your reactions and assumptions.

5. Deepen your child's symbolic exploration by providing toys and materials that allow them to expand on their play themes. For example, rescue vehicles can be offered if they frequently reenact saving scenarios.

6. As feelings emerge, empathize with the experience of the characters. Make comments like "Teddy seems really scared right now" or "The superhero is working hard to protect everyone."

7. If your child seems stuck in a repetitive, rigid play theme, gently offer an alternative perspective or plot twist. Play out a nurturing resolution to a typically chaotic story. Notice how your child responds to this challenge to their script.

Tips:

- Keep your observations and interpretations tentative and open to revision. Your child's play is a dynamic, evolving expression, not a fixed message.
- Avoid confronting your child directly about concerning themes. Let the play speak for itself, and trust that your child will work through the issues in their way as they feel safe.
- Discuss significant play patterns with other caregivers to gain additional insights and coordinate responses. Consider consulting with a play therapist for persistent distress or reenactments.

EXERCISE 3: SPORTSCASTER

Objective:

This activity helps parents provide a nonjudgmental, attuned presence by verbally reflecting on their child's play without interpretation or direction.

Materials:

- Open-ended toys
- Quiet, private space
- Patience and presence

Instructions:

1. Join your child's play session by asking if they would like you to watch them play and describe what you see. Explain that you will be a "sportscaster" sharing the highlights of their play.

2. Position yourself close enough to observe details but not so close that your child feels crowded or intruded upon. Orient your body to face your child and make occasional eye contact.

3. As your child plays, verbally reflect their actions, dialogue, and expressions using concise, descriptive statements. Avoid labeling feelings or motives. Use "you" statements instead of "I see."

Examples:

"You're stacking the red block on top of the blue block."

"The lion is saying 'Roar!' to the zebra."

"Your face is scrunching up as you mix the play dough."

4. Mirror the pace and tone of your child's play in your reflections. For fast, intense play, your voice might be more animated. For quiet, focused play, keep your voice soft and slow.

5. Resist the urge to praise, correct, or interpret your child's play. If they look to you for a response, nod or provide a simple affirmation like "I'm here, watching."

6. If your child invites you to join their play, ask how you can participate while still allowing them to direct. If they hand you a toy, describe how you are interacting with it.

7. When the play comes to a natural conclusion, provide a summary of what you observed, highlighting your child's creativity and focus. Thank them for letting you be their sportscaster.

Tips:

- Bite your tongue if you feel compelled to teach or problem-solve during play. Trust that your child knows what they need and will ask for help directly if desired.
- Practice observing play without narrating to build your capacity for silent attunement. Notice what thoughts and feelings arise for you as you witness.
- Expect your child to "dismiss" you at times to play independently. Honor this need for autonomy while remaining available nearby for connection. Your quiet presence is still valuable.

Remember, the goal of child-centered play techniques is not to arrive at a specific outcome or interpretation but to create a safe, accepting space for your child to explore, express, and integrate their experiences. By following your child's lead with curiosity and empathy, you send the message that their inner world is valid, valued, and understood. This secure base frees them to grow.

CHAPTER 6: UNLEASHING CREATIVITY THROUGH EXPRESSIVE ARTS

THE HEALING POWER OF ART, MUSIC, DRAMA, AND STORYTELLING

Close your eyes and think back to a time when you were bursting with big feelings - maybe excitement, fear, anger, or loss. How did you instinctively express those emotions? Did you doodle bold lines, dance with abandon, belt out a song, or act out an elaborate story? Chances are, you gravitated towards some form of creative expression, even if you didn't call yourself an "artist."

For children, the expressive arts are more than just fun pastimes - they are a vital outlet for making sense of life's joys and sorrows. When words fail or overwhelming experiences get stuck inside, the languages of art, music, drama, and storytelling offer a lifeline. Through painting, drumming, role-playing, or crafting tales, kids can release pent-up feelings, reframe challenges, rehearse solutions, and re-author their life stories.

Extensive research has documented the therapeutic benefits of expressive arts for children's mental health. Regular creative activities have been shown to:

- Reduce stress, anxiety, and depression symptoms
- Improve emotional regulation and impulse control
- Enhance self-awareness, self-esteem, and identity development
- Increase focus, flexibility, and problem-solving skills
- Foster social-emotional learning and empathy
- Build resilience and post-traumatic growth

By engaging multiple senses and tapping into the brain's right hemisphere, expressive arts bypass verbal defenses and access deeper wells of intuitive healing. They provide a safe container for kids to explore scary, confusing, or taboo topics at a symbolic distance. A 7-year-old grieving Grandpa's death might not want to talk about it directly but will bury and resurrect toys in the sand tray for weeks. An 11-year-old bullied at school might puppet a story of the ugly duckling's triumph.

The beauty of expressive arts is that there's no right or wrong way to do them. The process of creating is more important than the product. A child's tangled scribble or tuneless song is just as valuable as a museum-worthy masterpiece if it authentically represents their inner experience. This takes the pressure off parents to be "good at" art in order to help kids reap its benefits!

Some creative interventions that can target common emotional challenges for 6-11-year-olds:

Art:

- Feeling Portraits: Paint, draw, or collage a self-portrait depicting an intense emotion. Show where and how you experience that feeling in your body.
- Worry Dolls: Craft a small doll or figurine out of clay, yarn, or popsicle sticks. Whisper a worry to it, then place it under your pillow or in a special box overnight to "hold" the worry for you.

Music:

- Musical Mood Check-In: Choose an instrument that matches your current mood (e.g., fast drumming for anger, soft chimes for calm). Play it, then describe what the feeling sounds like.
- Lyric Rewrite: Take a familiar song and change the words to express your own experience or desired outcome (e.g., rewriting "Row, Row, Row Your Boat" to be about overcoming a fear).

Drama:

- Superhero Scenes: Create and act out a skit in which a superhero faces their kryptonite (i.e., a trigger or challenge) and practices their signature strength or power to defeat it.
- Feelings Charades: Take turns silently acting out an emotion or situation while others guess what it is. Then, discuss times you've felt that way and what helps.

Storytelling:

- Mixed-Up Fairy Tales: Tell a classic story (e.g., Three Little Pigs) from the perspective of a different character (e.g., the misunderstood wolf). Highlight their unique struggles, strengths, and desires.
- Alternate Ending Stories: Think of a book, show, or movie with a sad or scary ending. Rewrite or act out a new ending that feels more hopeful or empowering.

The key is to introduce these activities playfully and model nonjudgmental acceptance of whatever emerges. Provide a variety of open-ended materials (e.g., paints, clay, instruments, scarves, puppets) and basic prompts, then follow your child's lead. Focusing on sensory details and here-and-now experiences, rather than analyzing or interpreting, helps kids stay emotionally regulated and engaged.

As with any new coping strategy, expect that your child may need time and practice to feel comfortable with expressive arts. They may resist at first, fearing they're not "talented enough," or start strong, then get frustrated when their vision doesn't match their skills. Validate these anxieties while reiterating that the only goal is to express themselves authentically. Praise their bravery, effort, and unique creative choices to build intrinsic motivation.

Over time, you may be amazed at the depth of healing that unfolds through your child's artistic process. A story that starts with the hero small and alone and ends with a circle of supportive friends. A painting of a broken heart transforms into a vibrant garden. The same creativity that helps kids survive hard things becomes a renewable resource for crafting a brighter future. And as their most important witness and co-creator, you get a front-row seat to the magic.

ADAPTING EXPRESSIVE ARTS FOR YOUR CHILD'S UNIQUE NEEDS

Just as every child has a unique set of challenges and strengths, their pathway into creative expression will be equally individual. One size does not fit all when it comes to therapeutic arts - what soothes one kid's anxiety might overwhelm another's sensory system. The trick is to experiment with different modalities and meet your budding artists where they are.

Some general principles for adapting arts activities to your child's needs:

Developmental Level:

- Younger kids (6-8) may prefer more sensory-based, movement-oriented activities with simple themes (e.g., finger painting feelings, dancing like different animals).
- Older kids (9-12) can handle more advanced, symbolic prompts that encourage self-reflection (e.g., crafting a personal mascot or writing a song about their life story).
- Break complex tasks into smaller steps and provide structure/choices as needed.

Emotional Challenges:

- Anxiety: Focus on grounding, rhythmic, repetitive creative tasks (e.g., weaving, drumming, tracing mandalas). Gradually progress from soothing to gently expansive themes.
- Anger/Trauma: Provide safe ways to release intense feelings (e.g., pounding/sculpting clay, splatter painting, writing unsent letters). Balance with calming repair activities.
- Depression: Choose upbeat music, humor, and bright colors to lift the mood. Highlight characters' resilience in stories. Set modest goals and celebrate small wins.

Learning Differences:

- ADHD: Use novelty, movement, and multi-sensory elements to sustain focus. Keep directions short, visual, and specific. Allow wiggle breaks.
- Autism: Honor needs for predictability—preview plans, provide schedules, allow repetition of comforting motifs, and respect sensory differences regarding materials.
- Language Disorders: Emphasize visual/tactile modalities over verbal. Use simple words, songs, and stories with clear cause-effect sequences.

By tuning into your child's unique profile, you can adapt arts activities to optimize engagement and emotional regulation. If they're getting overstimulated by too many sensory inputs, scale back to one medium at a time. If they're struggling to initiate ideas, offer a menu of specific prompts to jump-start their imagination. If frustration is mounting, suggest a calming breath or silly wiggle break.

It's also important to follow your child's natural creative inclinations. Some kids will dive into painting with gusto, while others strongly prefer music or movement. Rather than forcing them to be "well-rounded," focus on the modalities that light them up. Lean into their favorite characters, themes, and materials as jumping-off points for therapeutic exploration.

That said, it can also be valuable to gently nudge kids outside their comfort zone at times. A child who defaults to drawing their feelings might find fresh insights by acting them out with puppets for one week. Variety sparks new neural pathways and coping strategies. Just be sure to frame it as a playful experiment rather than a command performance.

As you witness your child's creative process over time, you may start to notice symbolic themes that signal their core concerns, hopes, and inner resources. A child who repeatedly casts themselves as a trapped animal or a soaring bird may be grappling with the need for freedom and autonomy. One who keeps rewriting the ending of a tragedy into a victory may be cultivating seeds of post-traumatic growth.

Please resist the urge to overanalyze or quiz your child about the meaning of their creations. Instead, wonder aloud about the strengths the hero is discovering or how it might feel in their body to spread wings and fly. By staying curious about the emotional essence of their artwork rather than intellectualizing it, you create space for your child to find their healing metaphors.

Even more than the content of your child's creative work, your delighted attention is the real gift. Your enthusiastic presence as they finger-paint a swirl of feelings or belt out a ballad of bravery tells them that their inner world matters, that their voice deserves to take up space, and that their unique vision and style are strength in a culture that often squelches kids' creative instincts in favor of product and perfection, your unwavering appreciation is a radical act of love.

So dust off your old guitar, grab some pots and pans to drum on, and dive into the beautiful mess of expressive arts with your child! With a dash of silliness and a heaping spoonful of self-compassion, you may discover your inner artist yearning to come out and play. And that joyful, generative energy may be the most healing force of all in your family.

EXERCISE 1: FEELINGS PAINTING

Objective:

This activity encourages children to express and explore their emotions through abstract art, developing self-awareness and creative coping skills.

Materials:

- Paper or canvas
- Paint (tempera, acrylic, or watercolor)
- Brushes, sponges, or other painting tools
- Smock or old clothes for mess protection

Instructions:

1. Invite your child to think about a feeling they have experienced recently or one they find difficult to put into words. Examples might include joy, sadness, anger, calm, love, or fear.

2. Encourage them to imagine what that feeling would look like if it were a painting. What colors, shapes, lines, and textures would represent that emotion?

3. Provide a variety of paints and tools for your child to experiment with. Invite them to play with the materials and see what emerges rather than trying to make it look a certain way.

4. As your child paints, reflect on what you notice about their process. For example, "You're using a lot of red and making sharp, jagged lines" or "That blue color seems to be spreading softly across the page."

5. When the painting feels complete, ask your child to title their artwork with the feeling it represents. Display the painting in a special place as a visual reminder of their emotional expression.

6. Repeat the process with different emotions over time. Notice any patterns or changes in how your child represents certain feelings. Use the paintings as a springboard for discussing emotional experiences and coping strategies.

Tips:

- Model the activity by creating your feelings painting alongside your child. Share your process and interpretation with vulnerability.
- Offer a variety of painting surfaces (e.g., paper, cardboard, fabric) and tools (e.g., brushes, sponges, fingers) to keep the activity engaging over multiple sessions.
- Emphasize process over product. Reassure your child that there is no right or wrong way to depict an emotion. The goal is honest self-expression, not artistic perfection.

EXERCISE 2: PLAYLIST OF MY LIFE

Objective:

This activity helps children use music to express and regulate their emotions, capture significant memories, and share their inner world with others.

Materials:

- Paper and pen or digital playlist maker (e.g., Spotify, iTunes)
- Access to music library or streaming service
- Listening device (e.g., headphones, speakers)

Instructions:

1. Invite your child to create a playlist of 5-10 songs that represent important moments, relationships, or themes in their life. Please encourage them to think beyond their current favorite songs to music that captures their journey.

2. Provide prompts to help your child brainstorm meaningful tracks:

- A song that reminds you of a happy memory
- A song that helps you feel calm when stressed
- A song that reflects a challenge you overcame
- A song that makes you think of an important person
- A song that captures your hopes for the future

3. Help your child search for and select songs using your music library or a streaming service. Create a digital playlist or write down the tracklist.

4. Listen to the playlist together, pausing after each song to discuss what it means to your child. Ask open-ended questions like:

- What does this song make you think of?

- How do you feel when you hear this music?
- What memories or images come to mind?
- What do you like about the lyrics or melody?

5. Reflect on any themes or patterns you notice across the selected songs. Share your reactions and experiences with the music to deepen the emotional connection.

6. Brainstorm creative ways to share or expand on the playlist, such as:

- Creating album art that represents the overall mood or message
- Adding songs for other family members based on shared memories
- Making a music video or dance to accompany a particularly meaningful track
- Playing the songs as a soundtrack to a photo slideshow of your child's life

Tips:

- Validate all musical choices, even if they don't align with your taste. The goal is to understand and appreciate your child's perspective.
- Offer to make a playlist of your own to share with your child. Modeling vulnerability and creativity will encourage them to dig deeper.
- Consider making collaborative playlists as a family to capture your collective journey and strengthen your shared identity. Update the lists during key transitions or milestones.

EXERCISE 3: STORYBOOK ABOUT ME

Objective:

This activity helps children make sense of their experiences, celebrate their unique strengths, and share their self-narrative through creative writing and illustration.

Materials:

- Blank book or paper stapled together
- Drawing and coloring materials (e.g., crayons, markers, colored pencils)
- Stickers, photos, or other collage items (optional)

Instructions:

1. Offer your child a blank book and a variety of art materials. Explain that they will be creating a special storybook all about themselves and their life so far.

2. Help your child brainstorm ideas for their storybook by asking open-ended questions:

- What are some of your earliest memories?
- Who are the most important people in your life?
- What are your favorite things to do?

- What are some challenges you have faced and overcome?
- What makes you unique and special?
- What are your hopes and dreams for the future?

3. Encourage your child to write and illustrate their story in whatever way feels meaningful to them. They might create a literal timeline, a fictional tale based on real events, or a series of symbolic scenes.

4. As your child works on their book, offer support as needed with writing, spelling, or generating ideas. Avoid directing the content or critiquing the artwork. The goal is self-expression, not perfection.

5. When the book is complete, invite your child to share it with you and other trusted friends or family members. Listen attentively and reflect on the aspects of the story that move or inspire you.

6. Display the book in a special place and revisit it together over time. Notice how your child's self-narrative evolves as they gain new experiences and perspectives. Consider adding chapters during major life events or transitions.

Tips:

- If your child is resistant to drawing, suggest alternative forms of illustration like collage, photography, or using stickers and stamps.
- Be prepared for your child's story to include painful or difficult memories as well as joyful ones. Validate the full range of their experiences and emotions.
- Consider creating a parent version or family sequel to your child's book. Seeing their story in the context of a larger narrative can foster a sense of belonging and resilience.

EXERCISE 4: FAMILY DRAMA

Objective:

This activity helps families explore their roles, conflicts, and strengths through collaborative storytelling and improvisation, building empathy and flexible problem-solving.

Materials:

- Open space for movement and dramatic play
- Simple props and costumes (optional)
- Poster board or large paper for brainstorming

Instructions:

1. Gather your family and explain that you will be creating and acting out an improvised play that represents your family's dynamics and experiences.

2. Brainstorm key "characters" in your family, including individual members, shared values, typical conflicts, and sources of strength or resilience. Write these on poster board.

3. Decide on a "genre" or tone for your play, such as comedy, drama, or fairy tale. Consider framing challenges as an epic quest or a hero's journey to build creative distance.

4. Choose a "director" to set the scene and characters for the first improvised act. The director might say, "This scene is about the Smith family arguing over chores. Mom will play the role of Responsibility, Dad will play Fairness, Sister will play Frustration, and Brother will play Cooperation."

5. Act out the scene, with each person embodying their assigned role. Focus on expressing the underlying needs and feelings of the characters rather than reaching a specific resolution.

6. After the scene, discuss what you noticed from each character's perspective. Share what seemed realistic or insightful, as well as what felt exaggerated or incomplete in the portrayal.

7. Rotate directors and roles for each new scene, exploring different aspects of your family dynamics. Consider acting out both challenging past events and ideal future scenarios.

8. Conclude the drama by sharing appreciation for each other's contributions and insights. Identify any new understandings or possibilities that emerged through the imaginative play.

Tips:

- Treat this as adult-facilitated playful exploration rather than a therapeutic intervention. Keep the tone light and stop the drama if strong emotions arise.
- If certain members are reluctant to perform, invite them to be an "audience" and share reflections on what they observe.
- Consider recording or writing down key scenes and insights from your family drama. Revisit and build on the story over time as your relationships evolve.

Remember, expressive arts are a powerful medium for self-discovery, emotional healing, and relationship growth. By engaging your child's imagination through painting, music, storytelling, and drama, you open new pathways for communication and connection. Trust the process and let your inner artist out to play!

CHAPTER 7: FINDING BALANCE IN STRUCTURED VS. UNSTRUCTURED PLAY

THE ROLE OF FREE, IMAGINATIVE PLAY IN HEALING

In our outcome-driven society, it's easy to view unstructured play as frivolous - a waste of time that could be spent learning "useful" skills. But for children, open-ended, imaginative play is serious business. It's the canvas upon which they paint their inner world, test out budding abilities, and make sense of life's complexities. Free play is anything but frivolous - it's a vital vehicle for healing and growth.

Picture a child who recently moved to a new town, leaving behind beloved friends and familiar routines. In his self-directed play, he might build a cozy fort filled with favorite stuffed animals, an oasis of security amidst all the changes. Or he might pretend to be a brave explorer, charting new territory and making friends with strange creatures. Through metaphorical stories and sensory-rich experiences, he is metabolizing his grief and excitement, regaining a sense of control and competence.

This type of unstructured, symbolic play allows children to process charged experiences at their own pace in their unique language. They can take on roles and scenarios that would be too overwhelming to confront directly, diffusing their emotional charge through fantasy and repetition. A girl who witnessed a car crash might stage accidents between her toy vehicles over and over until the fearsome event feels more predictable and manageable. Each time, her play narrative might shift slightly as she experiments with causes, consequences, and solutions.

Extensive research confirms the healing power of imaginative play. Studies have found that a mere 30 minutes of daily pretend play can help children:

- Express and regulate intense emotions
- Develop a coherent sense of self and personal history
- Increase social skills like empathy, cooperation, and communication
- Improve problem-solving, divergent thinking, and cognitive flexibility
- Boost confidence, optimism, and a sense of agency
- Process and integrate stressful experiences
- Increase frustration tolerance and impulse control
- Build a repertoire of coping strategies and resilience

Far from being an escape from reality, imaginative play is the laboratory in which children alchemize challenges into opportunities for growth. Through roleplay and world-building, they can test out different ways of being, relating, and coping. Unbound by "real world" constraints, their brain is free to generate wildly creative solutions and narratives. Bit by bit, these playful experiments shape the architecture of their mind and expand their capacity to navigate life's inevitable ups and downs.

As a parent, your primary role in free play is to protect the conditions that allow it to thrive - time, space, open-ended toys, and a safe emotional climate. This means resisting the urge to jump in and direct the action, even when your child's play takes a dark or destructive turn. Barring any real safety risk, aim to be a calm, grounded presence, observing and reflecting rather than correcting or controlling.

This can be especially challenging when your child is working through painful experiences or exhibiting troubling behaviors in their play. It's natural to want to rush in and rewrite the ending or pepper them with questions about what their stories mean. But just as a caterpillar needs the struggle of emerging from its chrysalis to strengthen its wings, children need the freedom to grapple with life's hardships through play to build resilience. Trust that with enough time, space, and support, your child's internal wisdom will lead them toward healing narratives.

Your job is to be their safeguard and sounding board. Provide simple, unobtrusive sportscasting of their play - "The dinosaurs are fighting over the castle. There's so much roaring and crashing!" Reflect on any emotions you observe - "Teddy seems really scared hiding in that dark cave." And delight in any positive shifts - "Wow, the superheroes found a clever way to work together to save the day!" By holding up a mirror to your child's inner world, without judgment or agenda, you affirm their inherent creativity and strength.

Of course, in moments when your child is stuck in a negative loop or flooding with distress, it may be necessary to gently guide them towards more grounding or soothing themes. Introduce a comforting character, wonder aloud about a magic helper, or model some deep dragon breaths. The key is to drop these hints lightly, always returning leadership to your child's imagination. With practice, they will internalize the coping strategies you've seeded, a lasting bulwark against life's storms.

As your child learns to navigate their inner wilderness through free play, they will naturally seek you out as an attachment anchor. By being a haven and secure base, you give them the courage to dive deep, knowing they can surface to your calming presence as needed. This delicate dance between venturing and returning, creating and confiding, is the heart of play's power to heal. So settle in, marvel, and meet them with unconditional warmth whenever they need to come home to your love.

ADDING PURPOSEFUL STRUCTURE TO REINFORCE GOALS

For all its healing potential, free play is not a panacea. Some challenges call for a more targeted approach - one that breaks down complex skills into digestible practice sessions. That's where structured play comes in. By thoughtfully designing games and activities that isolate and rehearse specific abilities, you can give your child's emotional intelligence a focused boost.

Imagine a child who frequently lashes out at peers when feeling frustrated. In his unstructured play, you might notice themes of good guys vs. bad guys, winnowing losers, or explosive disasters. While processing these dynamics through fantasy is important, he may also benefit from step-by-step coaching on how to identify and tame his anger before it erupts. That's where structured games come in handy.

You might introduce a "Feelings Thermometer" game, where you take turns drawing Situation Cards (e.g., "Someone cut in front of you in line") and rating your anger level on a red-to-blue color scale. You can brainstorm calming strategies for each zone - deep breaths, positive self-talk, walking away - then role-play using them in sample scenarios. The repetition and simulation build his emotional vocabulary and impulse control.

Or take a child who has trouble seeing others' perspectives and communicating clearly. Her pretend play might be filled with one-sided dialogues or flat characters. To complement her imaginative explorations, you might play a structured "Social Detective" game where you take turns reading facial expressions and body language cues on Emotion Cards. By earning points for guessing others' feelings and needs, she gains practice in stepping outside her viewpoint. The gamified format keeps it light and engaging rather than a dreaded lecture.

Well-designed therapeutic games can target a range of social-emotional skills:

- Emotional awareness and expression (e.g., Feelings Charades, Mood Music)
- Empathy and perspective-taking (e.g., Guess My Intention, Mixed-Up Fairy Tales)
- Impulse control and problem-solving (e.g., Red Light/Green Light, Maze Craze)
- Coping and self-regulation (e.g., Calm-Down Scavenger Hunt, Yoga Pretzel)
- Communication and social skills (e.g., Talkabout, Fill Your Bucket)
- Flexibility and resilience (e.g., What's Another Way?, Bounce-Back Bingo)

The key is to balance didactic elements with plenty of playful, multisensory fun. A color-coded visual guide to coping strategies sticks better when each skill is linked to a goofy dance move or character. A turn-taking board game is more motivating when kids get to design their own wacky Challenge Cards. By weaving therapeutic content into absorbing, imaginative contexts, you harness kids' natural learning instincts.

When planning structured play, consider your child's developmental level, interests, and frustration threshold. A 6-year-old with a short attention span might thrive on simple, active games with clear rules and quick rewards. A 10-year-old wrestling with peer dynamics may dive into nuanced social dilemma discussions and complex cooperative projects. The sweet spot is a balance of achievable challenges and confidence-building wins.

As you introduce a therapeutic game or activity, provide an enticing hook that frames the target skill positively. Instead of "Let's practice sitting still," try "Want to learn some ninja breathing tricks to find your inner calm?" Support your child's autonomy by offering guided choices: "Do you want to be the Emotions Detective or the Body Language Bandit first?" Fuel their sense of competence with specific praise for effort and progress, not just perfect execution.

Although adult guidance takes a more central role in structured play, your child's agency is still paramount. Invite them to brainstorm variations on games, tailor content to their interests, and evaluate what works and what doesn't. Provide a predictable but flexible framework within which they can take ownership of the learning process. Through this collaborative approach, they internalize skills as part of their evolving identity, not just rules imposed from outside.

As your child gains fluency in naming emotions, swapping perspectives, bouncing back from upsets, and reaching out for support, celebrate these milestones with a silly victory dance or high-five ritual. Take time to reflect together on how their new strategies are making a difference in their day-to-day lives. Ask them what hidden superpowers they've discovered through all their hard work—and be sure to share your awe at their unique strengths.

With an artful mix of open-ended exploration and guided skill-building, play can be a transformative tool for growth. By knowing when to step back and follow your child's lead and when to gently scaffold specific competencies, you become an expert facilitator of their emotional education. As they stretch their creative muscles and master new coping tools, you'll be amazed at the resilient, resourceful protagonist they're becoming - both in the imagination and the real world.

EXERCISE 1: FOLLOW THE LEADER

Objective:

This activity helps family members practice flexibility, attunement, and creativity by taking turns leading and following in imaginative free play.

Materials:

- Open space for movement and play
- Simple props or toys (optional)

Instructions:

1. Choose a leader to start the imaginative play scenario. The leader might begin by saying, "Let's pretend we're explorers in a jungle!" or "I'm a chef in a busy kitchen!"

2. The leader begins moving and acting out their imagined scene, using body language, facial expressions, and simple dialogue. They may incorporate props or toys as part of the story.

3. The other players follow the leader's actions and words as closely as possible, mirroring their movements, emotions, and tone. They can add their creative details that fit the general theme.

4. After a few minutes, the leader can pass the role to another player by saying, "Follow [new leader's name]." The new leader then picks up the story where it left off and guides the group in a new direction.

5. Continue rotating leaders until each person has had a chance to guide the play at least once. Notice how the story evolves and transforms with each new perspective.

6. After the game, discuss what you enjoyed about each person's leadership style and imaginative choices. Reflect on how it felt to follow another's lead and adapt to their creative vision.

Tips:

- Encourage leaders to start with a general theme or setting but allow the story to emerge organically through play rather than planning it out in advance.
- Embrace silly, surreal, or unexpected twists in the story. The goal is creative expression and connection, not a coherent narrative.
- If a player feels stuck or unsure as the leader, offer gentle prompts or suggestions to help them find their footing. Emphasize that there is no "right" way to lead the play.

EXERCISE 2: GAME REMIX

Objective:

This activity encourages flexibility, problem-solving, and emotional expression by adapting familiar board games with new therapeutic rules and themes.

Materials:

- Board game of your choice (e.g., Monopoly, Candyland, Jenga)
- Paper and pencil for modifying rules
- Additional props or game pieces (optional)

Instructions:

1. Choose a board game that your family enjoys playing together. Gather the game materials and invite everyone to brainstorm ways to "remix" the game with a therapeutic twist.

2. Generate ideas for new rules or themes that promote emotional awareness, coping skills, or family connection. For example:

- In Monopoly, players share a self-care strategy or gratitude each time they pass "Go."
- In Candyland, certain colors represent different feelings, and players share a time they experienced that emotion when they landed in that space.
- In Jenga, players answer a relationship-building question or offer an appreciation before each turn.

3. Write down the new rules and any additional materials needed. Collaborate to refine the ideas and ensure everyone understands the modifications.

4. Play the remixed game, following the new rules and themes. Encourage players to be creative and expressive in their responses and actions.

5. After the game, debrief on what you noticed and enjoyed about the therapeutic version. Discuss any insights or challenges that arose through the modified play.

6. Consider rotating who gets to "remix" the game each time you play. Keep a running list of your family's favorite modifications and themes.

Tips:

- Choose themes that reflect your family's current needs or challenges. For example, if you're working on building trust, create rules that involve sharing vulnerabilities or offering support.
- Adapt the level of emotional depth to your child's developmental stage and comfort level. Start with lighter themes and gradually increase the intensity over time.
- Be willing to adjust or abandon rules that don't work in practice. The goal is to create a playful, meaningful experience, not to rigidly adhere to a predetermined structure.

EXERCISE 3: MOVE TO THE BEAT

Objective:

This activity promotes emotional attunement, nonverbal communication, and creative self-expression through a balance of structured and improvised dance.

Materials:

- Music player and speaker
- Playlist of diverse musical styles and moods
- Open space for movement

Instructions:

1. Create a playlist of songs that evoke a range of emotions and energy levels, from slow and gentle to upbeat and lively. Aim for a mix of familiar and new tunes.

2. Invite your family to gather in an open space where everyone has room to move freely. Explain that you'll be taking turns leading and following each other in dance to different songs.

3. Start the music and have one person begin dancing in their way, expressing the emotions and rhythms they hear in the song. Please encourage them to use their whole body and experiment with different movements.

4. After a minute, have the other family members join in by copying the leader's moves as closely as possible. Sync your breath and energy to theirs as you mirror their actions.

5. When the song changes, a new leader takes over and begins dancing in their style. The rest of the family follows their lead, adjusting to the new tempo and tone.

6. Continue rotating leaders with each new song, letting each person's unique self-expression emerge through their improvised moves. Notice how the group energy shifts and aligns with each leader.

7. End the dance session with a calming song and a group hug or squeeze. Take a moment to reflect on any emotions, sensations, or insights that arose through the movement.

Tips:

- Affirm all forms of creative expression, even if they feel awkward or unfamiliar at first. The goal is to embrace vulnerability and authenticity, not to perform or impress.
- If a family member feels self-conscious, offer the option to close their eyes or face away from others while dancing. Emphasize that there is no "right" way to move.
- Consider extending the activity by having each person choose a song that represents their current emotional state and sharing what the music means to them.

EXERCISE 4: BUILD-A-STORY

Objective:

This activity fosters collaboration, imagination, and flexible thinking by combining structured story prompts with open-ended creative play.

Materials:

- Story prompt cards (purchased or homemade)
- Toys, props, or costumes for acting out stories
- Recording device (optional)

Instructions:

1. Gather a variety of story prompt cards that include elements such as characters, settings, problems, and magical objects. You can purchase pre-made sets or create your own by writing ideas on index cards.

2. Invite your family to sit in a circle and draw a prompt card from each category (character, setting, problem, object). Read the selected prompts aloud to set the stage for the story.

3. Begin the story by having one person introduce the character and setting based on the prompts. For example, "Once upon a time, there was a shy unicorn living in a bustling city..."

4. Pass the storytelling to the next person, who adds a new plot point or challenge based on the problem card. For instance, "The unicorn desperately wanted to make friends but was afraid to approach anyone."

5. Continue rotating the storytelling, with each person building on the previous ideas and incorporating the magical object prompt when it fits. Encourage everyone to be creative and take the story in unexpected directions.

6. When the story reaches a natural conclusion or time runs out, reflect on the collaborative process. What did you enjoy about each person's contributions? What surprised or delighted you about the story?

7. If desired, act out favorite scenes from the story using toys, props, or costumes. Consider recording or writing down the full story to revisit and expand on later.

Tips:

- Adapt the prompt cards to your child's developmental level and interests. For younger children, use simple, concrete ideas and familiar themes.
- If a player gets stuck or goes off track, gently guide them back to the main storyline or suggest how to incorporate their idea.
- Encourage a balance of structure and spontaneity in the storytelling. The prompts provide a framework, but the real magic happens in the imaginative leaps between them.

Remember, the goal of balancing structured and unstructured play is to create a "just right" challenge that engages your child's creativity while providing a sense of safety and support. By flexibly alternating between leading and following, familiar and novel, planned and spontaneous, you help your child develop the resilience and adaptability needed to thrive in an ever-changing world. Trust your intuition and follow the fun!

CHAPTER 8: TAILORING PLAY TO YOUR CHILD'S DEVELOPMENTAL STAGE

MEETING YOUR SCHOOL-AGED CHILD WHERE THEY'RE AT

As any parent of a 6 to 12-year-old knows, the elementary years are a time of astonishing growth and change. In what seems like the blink of an eye, your pudgy preschooler transforms into a lanky tween with a quirky sense of humor and an unquenchable thirst for knowledge. Amidst all the intellectual leaps and social strivings, playtime remains a vital arena for your child to process the joys and perils of their expanding world.

To create a therapeutic play environment that truly meets your child's needs, it's essential to understand the developmental milestones they're navigating. While every child unfolds at their own unique pace, some common shifts in play behavior emerge as kids move through the school years:

Early School Age (6-8 years):

- Engage in elaborate fantasy play with complex storylines and character development
- Prefer cooperative play with peers, forming clubs and making up games with rules
- Develop a strong sense of fairness and loyalty, leading to frequent tattling and friend drama
- Enjoy collecting, sorting, and classifying objects based on concrete attributes
- Begin to grasp basic concepts of time, money, and categorization
- Still think in egocentric and magical terms, blurring fantasy and reality

Middle School Age (9-11 years):

- Shift towards more realistic, goal-oriented play that tests emerging skills and identities
- Engage in competitive games and sports with complex strategies and teamwork
- Form exclusive friend groups based on shared interests, with hints of cliquishness
- Develop a keener sense of self-consciousness and social comparison
- Grapple with moral dilemmas and existential questions in play themes
- Demonstrate increasingly abstract, logical thinking and problem-solving abilities

Knowing these general patterns can help you tailor play experiences to your child's sweet spot of challenge and mastery. In the early school years, your child may revel in dress-up and make-believe, so providing open-ended props and ample time for unstructured dramatization is key. As their social world expands, you might introduce collaborative games that reward cooperation over competition, like building a giant marble run or solving a mystery together.

As kids move towards the tween years, their play tends to become more grounded in reality, with an emphasis on tangible goals and products. They may pour their energy into perfecting a tricky skateboard move, writing and producing their skit, or mastering a complex board game strategy. This is a great time to offer activities that build on their developing logic and perspective-taking skills, like debating current events or role-playing social scenarios with nuanced characters.

Of course, every child's developmental trajectory is beautifully distinctive, shaped by their unique biology, experiences, and environment. A dreamy 10-year-old may still spend hours immersed in vivid fantasy worlds, while a scientifically-minded 7-year-old may prefer hands-on experiments to imaginative escapades. By tuning into your individual child's interests, abilities, and challenges, you can craft a play world that stretches but doesn't overwhelm them.

Some tips for developmentally attuned play:

- Offer a mix of familiar, comforting toys and novel, challenging activities to strike a balance between security and growth
- Break complex games or projects into achievable steps, providing just enough guidance to prevent frustration
- Use visual cues, concrete examples, and multisensory elements to make abstract concepts more tangible
- Encourage experimentation and creative problem-solving rather than focusing on "right" answers or perfect execution
- Validate the big feelings that come with growing up, from friendship woes to existential angst, through empathetic play characters and storylines
- Engage in sensitive role-play to practice navigating tricky social situations and expressing needs assertively
- Allow ample time for unstructured, child-led play to process learning and restore a sense of control

Above all, remember that your child's play is not meant to fit a cookie-cutter mold but to reflect their wonderfully weird and wise inner world. By accepting and celebrating their unique play preferences - even if they don't match the latest parenting manual - you permit them to grow at their own organic pace. So what if your 12-year-old still sleeps with a teddy bear or your 6-year-old prefers Shakespearean soliloquies to playing house? Embracing their developmental reality is the foundation for playful learning.

LEVERAGING YOUR CHILD'S NATURAL INTERESTS FOR ENGAGEMENT

Dinosaurs. Minecraft. Beyblades. Harry Potter. Whether your child is obsessed with prehistoric reptiles, addicted to a video game, or convinced they're secretly a wizard, chances are they have some intense passions that mystify and delight you. While it's tempting to view these fixations as distractions from the "real work" of therapeutic play, they are actually some of your greatest allies in capturing your child's engagement and cooperation.

Think of your child's unique fascinations as a powerful currency - an energy source you can harness to fuel their growth. By taking the time to understand what sparks their curiosity and makes them feel competent, you can design play experiences that piggyback on their natural motivations. Suddenly, the same child who claims to hate talking about feelings is eager to explore the emotional life of his favorite Pokemon character, and the kid who can't sit still for a board game is hyper-focused on beating her high score in a therapeutic video game.

Some ideas for integrating children's interests into therapeutic play:

- Use beloved stuffed animals or action figures as "co-therapists" to teach and model coping strategies

- Create a social story or comic book featuring a child's favorite character navigating a challenge they relate to
- Turn a repetitive video game action, like jumping or shooting, into a cue to practice a calm-down skill
- Design a board game based on a popular book series, with challenges and triumphs drawn from the plot
- Write and perform a skit in which treasured superheroes or villains work out conflicts and learn life lessons
- Adapt a classic game like Simon Says or Red Light/Green Light to feature commands from a child's cherished TV show
- Build a themed sensory bin or calm-down kit filled with toys and trinkets related to a special interest

The key is to enter your child's world with genuine curiosity and playfulness rather than co-opting their passions for your agenda. Get them talking about what they love most about their favorite game or character - the sense of mastery, the exciting storylines, the feeling of belonging to a fandom. Ask them to teach you the ins and outs of their most prized possessions, and really listen as they light up with expertise.

As you gain a deeper appreciation for your child's interests, you'll start to see natural connections to the skills and concepts you're aiming to reinforce. Maybe Minecraft is really about resourcefulness and resilience in the face of challenges. Maybe Pokemon is an allegory for appreciating individual differences and finding strength in diversity. By framing their existing fascinations in a growth-oriented light, you open up a whole new realm of learning that feels relevant and exciting to them.

Of course, you don't have to stretch to find a therapeutic tie-in for every obscure obsession. Sometimes, a lightsaber duel is just a lightsaber duel! But by honoring the things that light your child up in all their quirky glory, you create a foundation of trust and respect that primes them to take risks and tackle challenges in your presence. You communicate that their inner world matters and that growth can feel not just tolerable but actually tailored to their unique awesomeness.

Importantly, don't be afraid to get silly and surrender to your child's lead as you riff on their favorite themes. If they want to spend 20 minutes monologuing as a wisecracking turtle, roll with it! The more you can embrace the zany, nonlinear flow of their imagination, the more they'll let down their guard and allow you into the unfiltered corners of their psyche. It's in these spaces of joyful attunement that true healing and transformation often take root.

As you venture together into the uncharted territories of your child's mind, you may find your own inner 6-year-old or 12-year-old awakening in wonderful, surprising ways. You may rediscover a sense of wonder at the endless possibilities of play or a renewed compassion for the bumps and bruises of growing up. Honor that instinct to connect with your child in the language that feels most authentic to them - whether that's an elaborate fairy world or a gritty superhero battle.

In the end, the content of your child's interests is less important than the spirit of delight and discovery you bring to exploring them together. By following the twists and turns of their evolving obsessions with a warm, steady presence, you become their ultimate safe base for growth. So dust off your wizard's cloak, pick up a lightsaber, and let your child's passions be your guide into a galaxy of playful healing.

EXERCISE 1: PLAY PREFERENCE QUIZ

Objective:

This activity helps parents identify their child's unique play personality and preferences so they can choose developmentally appropriate activities that engage and challenge them.

Materials:

- Play Preference Quiz (see sample questions below)
- Pen or pencil
- Quiet space for reflection

Instructions:

1. Set aside 15-20 minutes of uninterrupted time to complete the Play Preference Quiz. Find a comfortable spot where you can reflect on your child's play habits and interests.

2. Answer each question on the quiz as honestly and specifically as possible, based on your observations of your child's recent play. Avoid comparing your child to others or selecting answers based on what you think they "should" prefer.

3. Tally your responses in each category to determine your child's primary play personality (e.g., Explorer, Creator, Competitor, Collaborator). Read the descriptions of each type to understand your child's unique play style and needs.

4. Reflect on how you can adapt your play invitations and environment to better suit your child's preferences. What types of toys, materials, or experiences might they enjoy most at their current stage?

5. Consider areas where your child might benefit from a gentle challenge or exposure to less preferred play styles. How can you gradually expand their comfort zone while honoring their natural inclinations?

6. Share your insights with other caregivers and your child, as appropriate. Invite them to offer their observations and ideas for supporting your child's play development.

Sample Play Preference Quiz Questions:

1. When given a choice, my child usually prefers:

  a) Active, physical games

  b) Creative, artistic activities

  c) Strategic, rule-based games

  d) Cooperative, social play

2. My child's favorite play materials tend to be:

  a) Open-ended, sensory-rich (e.g., sand, water, clay)

b) Imaginative, symbolic (e.g., costumes, figurines, puppets)

c) Structured, goal-oriented (e.g., puzzles, board games, sports equipment)

d) Interactive, collaborative (e.g., building sets, party games, science kits)

3. When facing a challenge during play, my child typically:

a) Persists independently, using trial and error

b) Invents creative solutions or adapts the rules

c) Seeks adult help or refers to instructions

d) Recruit peers to problem-solve together

4. My child's play interests and abilities seem to be:

a) Rapidly developing, with frequent leaps to new stages

b) Creatively evolving, with unique or advanced skills

c) Steadily progressing, with mastery of each level before moving on

d) Socially expanding, with a focus on shared experiences over solo achievement

Tips:

- Remember that play personalities are not fixed types but fluid preferences that can shift over time and across contexts. The goal is not to label your child but to understand and respond to their current needs.
- Look for ways to combine your child's preferred play style with other modes of learning and expression. For example, an Explorer might enjoy using natural materials to create an imaginative story (Creator), compete to build the tallest tower (Competitor) or lead a nature scavenger hunt with friends (Collaborator).
- Regularly update your understanding of your child's play personality as they grow and change. What engages them at age 4 may be quite different from what they need at age 8 or 12.

EXERCISE 2: STAGE-O-METER

Objective:

This activity helps parents evaluate the developmental fit of different play activities and toys so they can provide "just right" challenges that support their child's growth.

Materials:

- List of play activities or toys
- Paper and pen
- Developmental stage descriptions (see examples below)

Instructions:

1. Make a list of 10-15 play activities or toys that your child currently enjoys or that you are considering introducing. Aim for a mix of familiar favorites and novel ideas.

2. Create a "Stage-o-Meter" scale on a piece of paper with three sections labeled "Too Easy," "Just Right," and "Too Hard." Leave space to write examples under each heading.

3. Review descriptions of typical play skills and interests at your child's current developmental stage (e.g., early childhood, middle childhood, preadolescence). Note key milestones and characteristics.

4. For each activity or toy on your list, consider how well it matches your child's current developmental needs and abilities. Ask yourself:

- Does this play experience offer an appropriate level of challenge, or is it likely to be boring or frustrating?
- Does it tap into the types of play and learning that are most engaging at this stage?
- Is it accessible and safe for my child to use independently or with minimal support?

5. Place each item on the Stage-o-Meter scale based on your evaluation. Activities that are well-matched to your child's current stage go in the "Just Right" section, while those that seem too simplistic or advanced go in the "Too Easy" or "Too Hard" sections.

6. Review your completed Stage-o-Meter and look for patterns. Are there certain types of play that you need to offer more of? Are there beloved activities that your child may be outgrowing developmentally?

7. Use your insights to adjust your play environment and offerings over time. Aim to maintain a balance of "Just Right" challenges that engage your child's current abilities while gently stretching them towards new skills.

Example Developmental Stage Descriptions:

Early Childhood (3-5 years)

- Engages in imaginative, symbolic play with simple storylines and roles
- Enjoys sensory exploration and creative expression with art, music, and movement
- Builds fine and gross motor skills through active play and manipulation of objects
- Develops social skills through parallel and associative play with peers

Middle Childhood (6-9 years)

- Engages in elaborate, rule-based pretend play with ongoing narratives and characters
- Enjoys strategy games, puzzles, and problem-solving challenges
- Builds advanced physical skills through sports, dance, and outdoor adventures
- Develops close friendships and social groups through cooperative play and shared interests

Preadolescence (10-12 years)

- Engages in complex, imaginative play with themes of identity, morality, and social status
- Enjoys competitive games, intellectual pursuits, and creative hobbies
- Builds self-esteem and autonomy through mastery of valued skills and roles
- Develops social-emotional intelligence through intimate friendships and group dynamics

Tips:

- Remember that developmental stages are not rigid categories but fluid progressions that vary based on individual differences and cultural contexts. Use stage descriptions as a general guide, not a fixed prescription.
- Be willing to adjust your Stage-o-Meter ratings based on your child's actual engagement and enjoyment of an activity. They may surprise you with their ability to tackle a challenging game or their continued delight in a simple toy.
- Involve your child in evaluating the developmental fit of their play activities. Ask for their feedback on what feels too easy, too hard, or just right. Empower them to make informed choices about how they spend their playtime.

EXERCISE 3: TOY MATCHMAKER

Objective:

This activity helps parents curate a developmentally appropriate toy collection that supports their child's current play needs and interests.

Materials:

- Current toy and game collection
- Developmental toy lists or guides (see examples below)
- Storage bins or labels

Instructions:

1. Gather all of your child's current toys, games, and play materials in one area. Sort them into broad categories, such as puzzles, dolls, art supplies, etc.

2. Review developmental toy lists or guides that recommend age-appropriate playthings based on key milestones and skills. Look for reputable sources, such as educational or pediatric organizations.

3. Create a "Keep," "Store," and "Donate" system for evaluating each toy:

- Keep toys that match your child's current developmental stage and interests and are safe, durable, and engaging.
- Store: Toys that your child has outgrown developmentally but that may be enjoyed again by a younger sibling or friend in the future.
- Donate Toys that are no longer developmentally appropriate, interesting, or in good condition for your child or others.

4. Sort each toy into the appropriate category, involving your child in the decision-making process as much as possible. Discuss why certain toys are being kept, stored, or donated.

5. Organize the "Keep" toys in a way that makes them accessible and appealing to your child. Use storage bins, shelves, or labels to create a play space that invites exploration and engagement.

6. Make a list of any gaps in your toy collection based on your child's current developmental needs and interests. Consult toy guides or ask other parents for recommendations to fill those gaps.

7. Plan a regular toy rotation and evaluation system to keep your child's play space fresh and developmentally appropriate over time. Aim to introduce new challenges while honoring their enduring favorites.

Example Developmental Toy Lists:

Early Childhood (3-5 years)

- Blocks and construction sets
- Puzzles with 12-20 pieces
- Pretend play props (e.g., kitchen sets, doctor kits, dress-up clothes)
- Art materials (e.g., crayons, markers, play dough, collage supplies)
- Picture books and simple board games
- Riding toys and climbing equipment

Middle Childhood (6-9 years)

- Complex building sets and model kits
- Puzzles with 50-100 pieces
- Board games and card games with strategic rules
- Science and nature kits (e.g., magnets, microscopes, bug catchers)
- Craft and hobby supplies (e.g., beads, origami, knitting)
- Sports equipment and outdoor adventure gear

Preadolescence (10-12 years)

- Advanced construction sets and robotics kits
- Puzzles with 500+ pieces

- Strategy games and brainteasers
- Art and music supplies for creative expression
- Books and magazines on topics of passionate interest
- Outdoor equipment for exploring nature and taking safe risks

Tips:

- Choose toys that offer open-ended, creative play opportunities rather than single-purpose, close-ended activities. The best toys are "90% child, 10% toy."
- Look for playthings that grow with your child, offering new challenges and variations as they develop. Avoid trendy toys that quickly become boring or obsolete.
- Prioritize toys that encourage social interaction, physical activity, and intellectual curiosity. Limit passive entertainment that discourages real-world play and learning.
- Regularly involve your child in sorting and organizing their toy collection. This helps them build decision-making skills, letting-go capacity, and gratitude for what they have.

EXERCISE 4: PASSION PROJECT

Objective:

This activity helps parents plan play experiences that deepen their child's engagement with a topic of passionate interest, supporting their development of expertise and intrinsic motivation.

Materials:

- List of your child's current passions or intense interests
- Brainstorming materials (e.g., paper, whiteboard, mind-mapping app)
- Resources related to the chosen passion (e.g., books, websites, museums, mentors)

Instructions:

1. Make a list of your child's current passions, including any topics, activities, or characters that they are intensely interested in and spend significant time and energy exploring. These may be enduring fascinations or fleeting obsessions.

2. Choose one passion to focus on for this project, ideally something that has positive developmental potential and aligns with your family values. Discuss the choice with your child to gauge their enthusiasm and ideas.

3. Brainstorm a variety of play experiences that could deepen your child's engagement with this passion, such as:

- Reading fiction and nonfiction books on the topic
- Watching documentaries or educational videos
- Visiting museums, exhibits, or real-world locations related to the interest
- Interviewing experts or enthusiasts in the field
- Engaging in hands-on projects or experiments
- Creating art, music, or stories inspired by the passion

- Teaching others about the topic through presentations or demonstrations
- Participating in clubs, competitions, or online communities centered on the interest

4. Choose 3-5 play experiences from your brainstormed list that are feasible, affordable, and developmentally appropriate for your child. Aim for a mix of independent, guided, and social activities.

5. Create a plan for implementing each play experience, including any materials, resources, or support needed. Set realistic timelines and expectations, leaving room for your child's ideas and initiative.

6. Launch the Passion Project with your child, framing it as a special opportunity to dive deep into a beloved topic. Please encourage them to document their learning and discoveries through a project journal, scrapbook, or digital portfolio.

7. Regularly check in with your child to see how the project is going, offering support and encouragement as needed. Look for ways to extend and evolve the project based on their growing knowledge and skills.

8. Celebrate the completion of the Passion Project with a special event or showcase, such as a family presentation, community exhibit, or online sharing. Reflect on how the project has deepened your child's engagement and expertise.

Tips:

- Follow your child's lead in choosing and pursuing their passion. Please resist the temptation to steer them towards topics that you find interesting or impressive. Authentic enthusiasm is key.
- Look for ways to connect your child's passion with other areas of learning and development, such as reading, writing, math, science, or social studies. Point out how experts in the field use these skills.
- Encourage a growth mindset around the Passion Project, emphasizing effort, curiosity, and improvement over perfection or innate talent. Celebrate challenges and mistakes as opportunities to learn.
- Set boundaries around the Passion Project to ensure that it remains a joyful, intrinsically motivating experience rather than an overwhelming obligation. Prioritize play and process overpressure and product.

Remember, tailoring play to your child's developmental stage is an ongoing process of observation, experimentation, and adaptation. By staying attuned to your child's changing needs and interests, you can create a play environment that engages their current abilities while nudging them towards new growth. Trust your child's unique timetable and honor their path of playful learning.

Part 3: Cognitive-Behavioral Play Interventions

CHAPTER 9: EXPLORING THOUGHTS AND FEELINGS THROUGH PLAY

RECOGNIZING COGNITIVE DISTORTIONS IN PLAY THEMES AND NARRATIVES

As children play, they reveal a rich inner world of thoughts, beliefs, and expectations that shape their understanding of themselves and their place in the world. Through the characters they create, the stories they enact, and the themes they explore, children give voice to their deepest hopes, fears, and assumptions about how life works. As a parent, tuning into these play narratives can offer invaluable insights into your child's cognitive landscape – and help you spot patterns of thinking that may be holding them back.

One powerful lens for making sense of these patterns is the concept of cognitive distortions – habitual ways of interpreting information that are negatively biased, inaccurate, or overly rigid. These distortions are like fun-house mirrors that warp your child's perceptions of reality, leading to exaggerated emotional reactions and self-limiting beliefs. While all children (and adults!) engage in some degree of cognitive distortion, when these thinking traps become pervasive and go unchallenged, they can contribute to anxiety, low self-esteem, and a sense of helplessness.

Some common cognitive distortions that may show up in children's play include:

1. Overgeneralization: Making a broad, negative conclusion based on a single incident or piece of evidence. A child who repeatedly enacts stories where making one mistake leads to complete ruin or rejection may be overgeneralizing.

2. Catastrophizing: Blowing negative events out of proportion or assuming the worst-case scenario. A child whose play frequently features themes of destruction, inescapable danger, or irreparable loss may be catastrophizing.

3. Black-and-white thinking: Seeing things in stark, all-or-nothing terms with no middle ground. A child who creates characters who are either entirely good or entirely bad, with no complexity or nuance, may be engaging in black-and-white thinking.

4. Mind reading: Assuming you know what others are thinking or feeling without evidence. A child who often plays out scenes where other characters judge them harshly or plot against them may be mind-reading.

5. Emotional reasoning: Treating feelings as facts and letting them dictate beliefs about reality. A child whose play revolves around characters who believe they are unlovable or unworthy because they feel sad or anxious may be emotionally reasoning.

As you observe your child's play with curiosity and presence, notice if any of these distorted themes or narratives emerge repeatedly. Are the characters' reactions disproportionate to the situations they face? Do conflicts resolve in overly simplistic or fatalistic ways? Do certain self-critical messages or worst-case assumptions keep popping up across different stories?

When you spot a potential cognitive distortion in play, please resist the urge to jump in and correct it directly. Instead, use reflective narration to gently highlight the pattern and invite your child to examine it from a different angle. For example:

"It seems like every time Teddy makes a small mistake in this story, all the other animals completely reject him and say he's terrible. I wonder if there could be another way they might react?"

"I notice that whenever Princess Pea feels scared in this adventure, she tells herself that means something really bad is definitely going to happen, and there's nothing she can do. That's a pretty big leap from a feeling to a fact."

By putting words to these distorted narratives in a nonjudgmental, curious tone, you create space for your child to step back and question their assumptions. You model the metacognitive skill of observing one's thought patterns with healthy detachment and flexibility. And you open the door to playfully exploring alternative perspectives that can loosen the grip of cognitive rigidity.

In the next section, we'll explore some creative ways to use play to challenge and reframe these distorted thoughts, helping your child develop a more accurate and adaptive inner monologue. By bringing a spirit of curiosity, experimentation, and even silliness to the realm of self-talk, you empower your child to become the master of their mental landscape – one imaginative leap at a time.

PLAYFULLY CHALLENGING NEGATIVE THOUGHTS AND BELIEFS

Once you've tuned into the cognitive distortions that may be shaping your child's play narratives, the real fun begins! With a spirit of playful collaboration, you can help your child explore and experiment with alternative ways of thinking that are more accurate, balanced, and emotionally helpful. The key is to approach these thinking traps not as facts to be debunked but as ideas to be played with and perspectives to be broadened.

Here are some creative play activities you can use to gently challenge your child's negative thoughts and beliefs:

1. The "What Else" Game: When you notice a character engaging in a cognitive distortion, like catastrophizing or black-and-white thinking, press the "pause" button on the story and invite your child to brainstorm alternative explanations or outcomes. Use prompts like "What else could happen?" or "What's another way they could think about this?" Encourage wild, silly, and far-fetched ideas, emphasizing creativity over realism.

2. Thought Bubble Skits: Grab some dry-erase markers and a pack of sticky notes, and get ready to put on a meta-cognitive play! Invite your child to choose a character and a scenario where distorted thinking is leading to distress. Take turns writing down the character's self-talk on sticky notes and affixing them to the character like thought bubbles. Then, collaborate to come up with alternative self-talk that is more accurate, compassionate, or solution-focused. Act out the scenario with the new thought bubbles and notice how it changes the emotional tone and outcome of the story.

3. The "Shrinking Potion" Experiment: Cognitive distortions tend to inflate negative thoughts to overwhelming proportions, crowding out more balanced and hopeful perspectives. To playfully challenge this tendency, introduce a magic "shrinking potion" that has the power to reduce the size and intensity of the most daunting worries. Whenever your child's play features an exaggerated negative belief, whip out your imaginary potion bottle and invite them to take a pretend sip. As they drink, make a funny shrinking sound effect and use your hands to physically "shrink" the worry down to a more manageable size. Then, brainstorm ways the character can cope with this now tiny-sized challenge.

4. *The "Other Eyes" Telescope:* Cognitive distortions often stem from seeing situations through a narrow, self-focused lens. To help your child expand their perspective-taking skills, introduce a special telescope that allows them to see the world through other characters' eyes. Whenever a play narrative gets stuck in a one-sided, distorted view, pull out your pretend telescope and invite your child to peer through it from another character's vantage point. Ask curious questions like "What might this situation look like to them? What might they be thinking or feeling that we can't see?" This playful reframing exercise can help your child develop empathy, consider alternative interpretations, and challenge the assumption that their thoughts are the only valid ones.

5. *Courtroom Roleplay:* Set up a pretend courtroom where negative thoughts go on trial, with your child playing the roles of prosecutor, defense attorney, judge, and jury. Choose a specific distorted belief that comes up in their play, like "I'm no good at anything" or "Everyone hates me," and put it in the defendant's chair. Guide your child in gathering evidence for and against the belief, calling "witnesses" from their real-life experiences to testify. Please encourage them to cross-examine each piece of evidence, looking for exceptions, exaggerations, and alternative explanations. In the end, have the jury render a verdict on whether the belief is fully accurate or needs to be revised. This playful exposure to the process of disputation can help your child internalize the skills of flexible, critical thinking.

As you engage in these playful cognitive reframing activities, remember to keep the tone light, curious, and collaborative. The goal is not to convince your child that their thoughts are "wrong" but to help them discover for themselves that their thoughts are not fixed facts but changeable interpretations that can be examined and edited. Celebrate their creativity, bravery, and flexibility in considering new perspectives, and model your willingness to question and revise your assumptions.

With regular practice, these playful cognitive challenges can become a natural part of your child's inner dialogue, equipping them with the tools to catch and correct their distorted thinking in real-time. By learning to approach their mind with a spirit of openness, curiosity, and even humor, your child can develop the resilience and adaptability to navigate life's challenges with greater ease and self-compassion. By joining them in this imaginative journey of mental exploration, you deepen your ability to model and embody the very flexibility and perspective-taking you seek to nurture in them.

EXERCISE 1: THOUGHT BUBBLE TAG

Objective:

This activity helps children practice identifying and expressing their thoughts and feelings in a playful, physical way.

Materials:

- Open space to run around

- Optional: Thought/feeling bubble printouts or cards

Instructions:

1. Explain the rules of Thought Bubble Tag: One person will be "It" and try to tag the other players. When someone is tagged, they must freeze in place and say a thought or feeling they might have in that position.

2. Demonstrate the game by having the child tag you and then freezing in an exaggerated pose. Say a thought or feeling that matches your body language, such as "I feel so excited!" or "I'm thinking about ice cream."

3. Have the child take a turn being "It" and chasing you. Make silly poses and name a variety of thoughts and feelings when tagged to model the range of inner experiences.

4. Play several rounds of tag, switching roles and encouraging the child to freeze in different positions and express diverse thoughts and feelings. Validate all of their responses and show curiosity about their internal world.

5. For a variation, you can prepare thought/feeling bubble cards in advance and have the tagged person draw one from a bowl to share. This can help prompt ideas and expand emotional vocabulary.

6. After playing, debrief with the child about what it was like to notice and share their thoughts and feelings on the spot. Highlight any patterns or insights you observed, such as how their body language matched their inner experience.

Tips:

- Adapt the pace and physicality of the game to your child's energy level and abilities.
- Model vulnerability by sharing a mix of comfortable and uncomfortable thoughts and feelings.
- Emphasize that all thoughts and feelings are valid and welcome in the game.

EXERCISE 2: DISTORTION DETECTIVE

Objective:

This activity helps children learn to recognize and challenge common cognitive distortions in media and daily life.

Materials:

- Age-appropriate books, shows, or movies that demonstrate cognitive distortions
- Detective props (e.g., magnifying glass, notepad, trench coat)
- List of common cognitive distortions and their definitions

Instructions:

1. Introduce the concept of cognitive distortions as "sneaky thoughts" that can make situations seem worse than they are. Share a few examples, such as all-or-nothing thinking or jumping to conclusions.

2. Present the idea of being a "Distortion Detective" who hunts for these tricky thoughts in stories or real life. Put on detective props and adopt a playful, curious tone.

3. Choose an age-appropriate book or show and read/watch it together, pausing whenever you spot a potential cognitive distortion. Ask the child to identify which distortion it might be and why.

4. When distortion is named, brainstorm alternative perspectives or thoughts that could be more accurate or helpful. Encourage the child to think like a detective and look for evidence that challenges the distortion.

5. Take turns being the lead detective and the assistant so that the child has a chance to guide the process. Celebrate each time a distortion is spotted and an alternative is found.

6. Extend the activity to real-life situations by sharing examples of distortions from your thoughts or experiences. Model how to catch and challenge them in the moment.

7. After playing, reflect on what the child learned about common cognitive traps and how to reframe them. Discuss how they can use their detective skills in daily life to manage tricky thoughts.

Tips:

- Start with simple, clear examples of distortions and gradually move to more subtle or complex ones.
- Use humorous examples or roleplay to keep the activity light and engaging.
- Praise the child's effort and insight rather than just the accuracy of their answers.

EXERCISE 3: SILVER LINING SPOTLIGHT

Objective:

This activity helps children build resilience and optimism by practicing finding the positives in challenging situations.

Materials:

- Flashlight or spotlight prop
- Optional: Silver lining tokens or stickers

Instructions:

1. Introduce the concept of a silver lining as the positive side or opportunity in a difficult situation. Share an example from your own life, such as "I missed the bus, but I got some extra exercise walking and saw a beautiful sunrise."

2. Present the Silver Lining Spotlight game, where players take turns sharing a challenge or disappointment and then "shining a light" on the potential bright side.

3. Model the activity by sharing a kid-friendly challenge, then passing the flashlight to the child and encouraging them to find a silver lining. Offer hints or prompts if needed, but let them generate their ideas.

4. Switch roles and have the child share a challenge, then guide you to find the positive. Ham it up as you search for the silver lining, making it a playful and engaging process.

5. Continue taking turns, with each person sharing a challenge and the other spotlighting the opportunity. Validate the child's feelings about the initial challenge while still encouraging a resilient mindset.

6. Consider awarding silver lining tokens or stickers for each one found to reinforce the skill. Collaborate to think of creative ways to cash in the tokens, such as for a special privilege or a silly family dance party.

7. After playing a few rounds, debrief on how it felt to look for the positives and what strategies were most helpful. Brainstorm how to remember this skill in the face of future disappointments.

Tips:

- Use age-appropriate examples and keep a quick, lighthearted pace to maintain engagement.
- Model persistence and creativity if the silver linings aren't immediately obvious.
- Emphasize that finding a silver lining doesn't negate the initial challenge or feeling but can help us cope and move forward.

EXERCISE 4: MISTAKE-MAKING CONTEST

Objective:

This activity helps children embrace mistakes as opportunities for learning and growth while challenging perfectionism.

Materials:

- Various materials for making playful "mistakes," such as:
- Paper and art supplies for drawing imperfect pictures
- Building blocks or LEGOs for creating lopsided structures
- Puzzles or games that can be played "wrong"
- Silly props or costumes for acting out exaggerated errors

Instructions:

1. Introduce the idea of a Mistake-Making Contest, where the goal is to make the most creative, courageous, and unexpected mistakes. Emphasize that in this game, mistakes are celebrated and learned from, not feared or avoided.

2. Model the activity by intentionally making a mistake, such as drawing a silly face with mismatched features or building a tower that tilts and falls. Exaggerate your reaction and "celebrate" the error with laughter and self-compassion.

3. Invite the child to take a turn making their own playful mistake using the available materials. Encourage them to think outside the box and not worry about doing it "right."

4. When a mistake is made, have the child share what they learned or discovered from the experience. Highlight the creativity, risk-taking, or problem-solving skills they demonstrated.

5. Take turns making and celebrating mistakes, with each person trying to outdo the other in terms of silliness or innovation. Keep the tone light and energetic, with lots of laughter and playful banter.

6. For an extra challenge, have each person intentionally make a specific type of mistake, such as in drawing, building, singing, or acting. See who can come up with the most imaginative or unexpected way to "fail."

7. After the game, debrief on how it felt to embrace mistakes and what insights were gained. Discuss how this mindset can be applied to real-life challenges or learning experiences.

Tips:

- Model self-compassion and a growth mindset by narrating your mistake-making process.
- Praise the child's effort, creativity, and resilience rather than the outcome of their mistakes.
- Adapt the activity to your child's interests and abilities, choosing materials that are engaging and appropriately challenging.
- If the child becomes frustrated or self-critical, gently remind them of the game's purpose and model how to reframe the mistake as a learning moment.

With these fun and meaningful exercises, children can learn to explore their thoughts and feelings, challenge cognitive distortions, and embrace mistakes as opportunities for growth. By approaching these skills through play, you create a safe and engaging environment for children to develop self-awareness, resilience, and a positive mindset.

CHAPTER 10: COPING AND PROBLEM-SOLVING THROUGH PRETEND PLAY

MODELING HELPFUL SELF-TALK AND COPING STATEMENTS

Imagine your child is playing with their favorite stuffed animal, and they encounter a frustrating obstacle in their make-believe world. Maybe the stuffed puppy can't seem to climb the block tower, or the teddy bear keeps stumbling in the pretend school race. How the child navigates this challenge in their play narrative can offer a powerful window into their real-life coping strategies and inner dialogue.

As parents, we have a unique opportunity to use pretend play as a vehicle for modeling and reinforcing helpful self-talk and coping statements. By voicing these messages through the characters in our child's play, we can gently plant the seeds of resilience, self-compassion, and a growth mindset—all in a way that feels natural, engaging, and developmentally appropriate.

So, what does this look like in practice? Let's say you're playing with your child and their stuffed puppy, and the puppy is struggling to climb the block tower. You might have the puppy voice a coping statement like:

"Wow, this tower is really tall and tricky to climb! But I know I can keep trying and do my best. It's okay if I don't get it right away – that's how I learn and get stronger."

Or let's say the teddy bear is feeling discouraged after stumbling in the pretend race. You might have the bear say something like:

"Oops, I tripped and fell behind in the race. That feels frustrating and disappointing. But I'm proud of myself for running the whole way and not giving up. Maybe next time I can practice more and see if I improve."

Notice how these statements acknowledge the difficulty of the situation while also emphasizing the character's ability to cope and persevere. They model self-compassion in the face of setbacks and reframe challenges as opportunities for growth and learning.

Some other helpful self-talk and coping statements you might weave into pretend play include:

- "This is tough, but I can handle it."
- "I'm feeling overwhelmed right now. I'm going to take a deep breath and break this down into smaller steps."
- "It's okay to feel frustrated when things don't go my way. I can safely express my feelings and then let them go."
- "Mistakes are part of learning. I can be kind to myself and keep trying."
- "I don't have to be perfect. I'm doing my best, and that's what matters."
- "When something is hard, that means I'm growing my brain!"

The key is to voice these statements in a way that feels authentic and attuned to your child's play scenario. Rather than lecturing or instructing, aim to model the language in a subtle, organic way. Please pay attention to your child's reactions and build on their ideas and interests.

You can also invite your child to brainstorm their coping statements for their characters. Ask open-ended questions like:

- "Hmm, that looks like a tricky situation for the puppy. What do you think he could say to himself to feel better and keep trying?"
- "I wonder how the bear is feeling after falling in the race. What kind words could we give him to help him feel proud of his effort?"

By encouraging your child to generate helpful self-talk, you empower them to become active agents in their own emotional regulation and resilience-building.

Over time, as your child hears these coping statements modeled repeatedly in their pretend play, they will start internalizing them as their inner dialogue. The language of resilience, self-compassion, and growth mindset will become increasingly automatic, guiding their real-life responses to frustration and setbacks.

PRACTICING PROBLEM-SOLVING STEPS THROUGH ROLE PLAY

In addition to modeling helpful self-talk, pretend play offers a rich opportunity to practice and reinforce problem-solving skills. By setting up imaginative scenarios that mirror real-life challenges and guiding your child through a step-by-step problem-solving process, you can help them build a robust toolkit for navigating life's inevitable obstacles with flexibility, creativity, and confidence.

One simple but powerful framework for problem-solving involves the following steps:

1. Identify the problem: What is the specific challenge or obstacle the character is facing?

2. Brainstorm solutions: What are some possible ways the character could address this problem? Encourage your child to generate multiple ideas, even if they seem silly or far-fetched.

3. Evaluate consequences: For each potential solution, consider the likely outcomes and consequences. Which ones seem most feasible and effective?

4. Make a plan: Choose one solution to try out and break it down into concrete steps. What will the character need to do first, second, and third?

5. Try it out: Have the character enact the plan in the pretend scenario. What happens as a result?

6. Reflect and adjust: After trying out the solution, encourage your child to reflect on how it went. Did it work as expected? If not, what could the character try differently next time?

Here's how you might guide your child through this process in a pretend-play scenario:

Let's say your child is playing with their stuffed animals, and a conflict arises between the lion and the giraffe over sharing a toy car.

1. Identify the problem:

"Uh oh, it looks like Lion and Giraffe both want to play with the same car at the same time. That's a tricky problem!"

2. Brainstorm solutions:

"Hmm, what do you think they could do to solve this problem? Maybe they could take turns driving the car or find another toy to play with together. What other ideas do you have?"

3. Evaluate consequences:

"Let's think about what might happen if they try taking turns. How do you think Lion would feel about waiting for his turn? What about if they played with a different toy instead? Which solution do you think would work best?"

4. Make a plan:

"Okay, so it sounds like you think taking turns might be a good solution. How could they make that happen? Maybe Lion could drive the car for 5 minutes while Giraffe cheers him on, and then they switch?"

5. Try it out:

Encourage your child to act out the turn-taking plan with the stuffed animals.

6. Reflect and adjust:

"So how did that turn-taking plan work out for Lion and Giraffe? Did they both get a chance to play with the car? Is there anything they might do differently next time to make the turn-taking even smoother?"

As you guide your child through this problem-solving process in their pretend play, remember to keep the tone curious, collaborative, and nonjudgmental. Please resist the urge to jump in with your solutions; instead, draw out your child's ideas and empower them to evaluate outcomes. If a solution doesn't work out as planned, reframe it as an opportunity to learn and innovate.

Some other everyday problem scenarios you might explore through pretend play include:

- Resolving a disagreement with a friend on the playground
- Completing a challenging homework assignment
- Navigating a change in routine or schedule
- Coping with disappointment when plans fall through
- Handling big feelings like anger or frustration in a healthy way

For each scenario, guide your child through the step-by-step problem-solving process, inviting their creativity and perspective-taking along the way. Praise their effort, flexibility, and persistence rather than focusing on the specific outcome.

By rehearsing these problem-solving skills repeatedly in the safe, low-stakes context of pretend play, your child will internalize them as a go-to strategy for navigating real-life challenges. They will develop a sense of self-efficacy and resourcefulness, trusting in their ability to find solutions even when the path forward is unclear.

Even more importantly, by engaging in this collaborative problem-solving process with you, your child will absorb the deeper message that they are not alone in facing life's obstacles. They will know that they have a caring, supportive ally who believes in their capacity to handle hard things and will guide them with wisdom and compassion.

And who knows – as you join your child in flexing your problem-solving muscles in the world of make-believe, you may discover some playful new strategies to apply in your grown-up life as well! After all, the power of imagination and creative thinking knows no age limit.

So go forth and let your pretend play be a joyful laboratory for building your child's resilience, one stuffed animal scenario at a time. With each silly skit, each zany brainstorm, and each triumphant resolution, you are nurturing the skills and mindset they need to navigate life's challenges with confidence, adaptability, and even a dash of humor.

And know that by showing up for your child in these playful problem-solving moments. You are giving them a priceless gift: the deep knowing that they are capable, supported, and loved beyond measure – no matter what obstacles come their way.

EXERCISE 1: COPING KIT SCAVENGER HUNT

Objective:

This activity helps children identify and practice using various coping strategies through a fun, hands-on scavenger hunt.

Materials:

A variety of items that can represent coping tools, such as:

- Stress balls or fidget toys for physical relaxation
- Calming images or nature sounds for visualization
- Journals or art supplies for expressive processing
- Favorite books or stuffed animals for comfort and distraction
- Bubbles or pinwheels for deep breathing
- Phone or device for calling a support person

Instructions:

1. Introduce the concept of a coping kit as a collection of tools and strategies that can help us feel better when we're stressed, anxious, or upset. Share examples of items that might go in a coping kit.

2. Present the Coping Kit Scavenger Hunt challenge, where the goal is to find or create as many coping tools as possible within a set time limit. Explain that for each item found, the player must also demonstrate how to use it for relaxation or stress relief.

3. Define the boundaries for the scavenger hunt, such as specific rooms or areas of the house/yard. Set a timer for an appropriate length (e.g., 15-20 minutes) and have the child begin searching.

4. As the child finds each item, have them bring it to you and explain how it could be used as a coping tool. Offer praise and guidance as needed while encouraging creative thinking.

5. If the child is struggling to find enough items, offer hints or suggestions for everyday objects that could be repurposed for coping (e.g., a smooth rock for grounding a soft blanket for comfort).

6. When the timer goes off, have the child gather all their coping tools and lay them out in one place. Review each item together and discuss when and how it might be most helpful.

7. Help the child assemble their finds into a special coping kit that can be easily accessed when needed. Decorate a box or bag to store the kit and keep it in a safe, comforting place.

8. After the activity, brainstorm additional coping strategies that might not have physical representations, such as positive self-talk, asking for help, or visualizing a peaceful scene. Add these ideas to the kit as reminder cards.

Tips:

- Tailor the scavenger hunt to your child's age and interests by choosing items that are developmentally appropriate and personally meaningful.
- Model using the coping tools yourself and share personal examples of when different strategies have worked for you.
- Encourage regular practice with the coping kit items, even when the child is not actively distressed, to build comfort and mastery.

EXERCISE 2: PUPPET PROBLEM-SOLVING

Objective:

This activity helps children practice identifying problems and brainstorming solutions through the playful, projective medium of puppet roleplay.

Materials:

- Several puppets or stuffed animals of different characters
- Optional: Craft materials for creating simple stick puppets (popsicle sticks, construction paper, markers, glue)

Instructions:

1. Introduce the concept of problem-solving as a way to deal with challenges or conflicts in a calm, constructive manner. Share the basic steps: 1) Identify the problem, 2) Brainstorm solutions, 3) Evaluate and choose a solution, 4) Try it out and adjust as needed.

2. Present the Puppet Problem-Solving activity, where the goal is to help the puppet characters work through various dilemmas using the problem-solving steps. Explain that the child will get to play one puppet while you play the other.

3. Choose a relevant scenario to act out with the puppets, such as a disagreement over sharing toys, a frustrating task, or a change in routine. Start the scene by having your puppet express the problem in a clear, concise way.

4. Have the child's puppet respond with empathy and validate the other character's feelings. Encourage them to ask clarifying questions to fully understand the problem.

5. Together, brainstorm potential solutions to the problem through the puppet dialogue. Encourage the child to generate multiple creative options without judging them yet. Model thinking out loud and building on each other's ideas.

6. Have the puppets evaluate the pros and cons of each solution, considering factors like fairness, safety, and practicality. Guide the child in choosing a solution to try, emphasizing that there may be multiple good options.

7. Act out the chosen solution with the puppets, having them work through any challenges or adjustments needed. Model flexible thinking and persistence.

8. Reflect on the process and outcome of the puppet problem-solving. What worked well? What could be done differently next time? Celebrate the characters' efforts and creativity.

9. Repeat the activity with different scenarios and puppet combinations. Encourage the child to generate their problem ideas based on real-life experiences.

Tips:

- Use humorous voices and exaggerated reactions with the puppets to keep the activity engaging and lighthearted.
- If the child gets stuck in the problem-solving process, offer hints or prompts through your puppet character, such as "I wonder if there's a way we could take turns?" or "What would happen if we asked an adult for help?"
- Connect the puppet scenarios to real-life situations and encourage the child to practice applying the problem-solving steps in their conflicts or challenges.

EXERCISE 3: CALMING CHARACTER CHARADES

Objective:

This activity helps children learn and practice various coping strategies through fun, active roleplay.

Materials:

- List of coping strategies or calming activities
- Timer
- Optional: Props or costume elements to represent each strategy

Instructions:

1. Introduce the concept of calming strategies as ways to relax our bodies and minds when we feel stressed, anxious, or overwhelmed. Brainstorm a list of specific strategies, such as deep breathing, progressive muscle relaxation, visualization, mindfulness, physical exercise, or creative expression.

2. Write each strategy on a separate slip of paper and put them in a bowl or hat. Explain the rules of Calming Character Charades: Players will take turns drawing a strategy and acting it out without words while the other players try to guess what it is.

3. Model the first round by drawing a strategy and silently demonstrating it with exaggerated actions and facial expressions. Encourage the child to observe closely and shout out their guesses.

4. Once the strategy is correctly identified, have everyone practice it together, with you leading and the child following along. Offer any necessary guidance or modifications.

5. Switch roles and have the child draw and act out the next strategy. Offer praise and encouragement for their creative portrayal and effort.

6. Continue taking turns until all the strategies have been demonstrated and practiced. Keep the pace lively and the tone playful, with lots of laughter and interaction.

7. For an added challenge, introduce a time limit for each charade (e.g., 30 seconds) and keep a score of how many strategies are guessed correctly within the time frame.

8. After the game, reflect on which strategies felt most natural or effective for each player. Discuss how and when to use these calming tools in real life, and brainstorm any additional strategies to add to the list.

Tips:

- Adapt the difficulty of the strategies to the child's age and familiarity. Start with simple, concrete techniques and gradually introduce more abstract or complex ones.
- Use props or costume elements to make the charades more engaging and memorable. For example, use a feather to represent deep breathing or a yoga mat for stretching.
- Model non-judgmental attitudes and self-compassion throughout the activity, emphasizing that calming strategies are personal and may take practice to master.

EXERCISE 4: OBSTACLE COURSE

Objective:

This activity helps children practice problem-solving and coping skills in a fun, physical challenge course.

Materials:

Various obstacles or challenges, such as:

- Pillows or cushions to represent "frustration rocks."
- Hula hoops or jump ropes represent "worry waves."
- Tunnels or cardboard boxes to represent "anxiety caves."
- Balls or beanbags to represent "angry energy."
- Signs or labels for each obstacle, listing a specific problem-solving or coping strategy.
- Timer or stopwatch.

Instructions:

1. Set up an obstacle course in a safe, open area, using various materials to create different physical challenges. Label each obstacle with a sign that describes a specific problem-solving or coping skill, such as "Take deep breaths," "Ask for help," "Break it down into steps," or "Find the positive."

2. Explain the rules of the Obstacle Course: Players must navigate through each challenge while practicing the corresponding skill. The goal is to complete the course as quickly as possible while demonstrating effective problem-solving and coping strategies.

3. Model the first round by verbally narrating your thoughts and actions as you go through the course. For example, "I'm feeling frustrated by these big rocks, so I'm going to take some deep breaths and think of a plan." Demonstrate how to use the labeled strategies at each obstacle.

4. Time the child as they complete the course, offering encouragement and guidance as needed. If they struggle with a particular obstacle or skill, provide hints or model it again.

5. After the first round, have the child reflect on which strategies worked well and which were more challenging. Brainstorm any modifications or new strategies to try in the next attempt.

6. Run the course several more times, encouraging the child to beat their previous time while still practicing effective problem-solving and coping skills. Offer praise and high-fives for effort and improvement.

7. For an added challenge, create a "mystery obstacle" at the end of the course, where the child must generate their own problem-solving or coping strategy to overcome it. Celebrate their creativity and resilience.

8. After the activity, debrief on how the problem-solving and coping skills used in the course could be applied to real-life challenges. Discuss any takeaways or insights gained from the experience.

Tips:

- Adjust the difficulty of the obstacles and skills to the child's age and abilities. Allow them to help design or set up the course to increase engagement and ownership.
- Use visual aids or demonstrations to explain each skill in addition to the written labels. Consider adding fun sound effects or music to enhance the playful atmosphere.
- Encourage the child to use positive self-talk and growth mindset language throughout the course, such as "I can do this" or "Mistakes help me learn."

EXERCISE 5: WHAT WOULD YOU DO?

Objective:

This activity helps children generate and practice problem-solving strategies for various hypothetical challenges.

Materials:

- Scenario cards describing age-appropriate problems or dilemmas
- Pencil and paper for brainstorming

- Optional: Props or costumes for role-playing

Instructions:

1. Introduce the What Would You Do? game, where players take turns drawing scenario cards and brainstorming solutions to the described problems. Explain that the goal is to think creatively and flexibly, considering multiple perspectives and possibilities.

2. Create a set of scenario cards that depict a range of age-appropriate challenges, such as:

- You forgot your homework at home, and the teacher is collecting it now.
- Your friend is playing with someone else at recess, and you feel left out.
- You accidentally broke your sibling's toy, and they are crying.
- The power went out, and you can't use your electronic devices.

3. Have the child draw the first card and read the scenario aloud. Ask probing questions to fully understand the problem, such as "How do you think the character is feeling?" or "What might happen if they don't solve this problem?"

4. Together, brainstorm potential solutions to the scenario, writing down each idea on a separate piece of paper. Encourage the child to think outside the box and consider unconventional approaches.

5. Review the brainstormed solutions and discuss the pros and cons of each. Have the child choose one or two solutions to act out, using props or costumes if desired.

6. Role-play the scenario and chosen solution(s), with you playing the other characters involved. Offer feedback and guidance as needed while keeping the tone playful and encouraging.

7. After acting out the scenario, reflect on how the solution(s) worked and whether any adjustments could be made. Discuss how the child might apply similar problem-solving strategies in their own life.

8. Repeat the process with additional scenario cards, taking turns brainstorming and acting out solutions. Celebrate creative and effective ideas while emphasizing that there are often multiple ways to approach a problem.

9. Conclude the activity by discussing common problem-solving themes or strategies that emerged across the scenarios. Brainstorm ways to practice and apply these skills in real-life situations.

Tips:

- Use humor and imagination in the brainstorming process to make it more engaging and memorable. Encourage silly or exaggerated solutions alongside more realistic ones.
- Tailor the scenarios to the child's specific experiences and challenges, such as social situations, academic tasks, or family dynamics. Allow them to generate their scenario cards as well.
- Model flexible thinking and persistence throughout the activity, showing that it's okay to try multiple approaches or adjust course when needed.
- Debrief after each scenario to reinforce learning and application. Ask questions like "What did you learn from this situation?" or "How could you use this strategy in your own life?"

CHAPTER 11: PLAYING THROUGH WORRIES AND FEARS

CREATING GRADUAL EXPOSURE HIERARCHIES THROUGH PLAY

Imagine for a moment that you're afraid of swimming. The thought of entering the water fills you with dread, and you worry that you'll sink or struggle to breathe. Now imagine that a well-meaning friend, in an effort to help you conquer this fear, throws you into the deep end of a pool without warning. Chances are, you'd emerge from that experience even more terrified of swimming and less trusting of your friend's support.

Now imagine instead that your friend invites you to sit by the edge of the pool and dangle your feet in the shallow end. As you acclimate to the sensation of the water and build confidence, they gradually encourage you to wade in deeper, offering reassurance and guidance along the way. With each small, achievable step, you start to challenge your fears and expand your comfort zone until, one day, you find yourself swimming with ease and joy.

This is the essence of gradual exposure therapy – a powerful approach for helping children overcome anxiety and phobias by facing their fears in a stepwise, playful manner. By breaking down a feared situation into manageable chunks and engaging with them repeatedly through play, children can desensitize their worries and build a sense of mastery and self-efficacy.

The first step in using gradual exposure play is to collaborate with your child to create a playful "fear ladder" or hierarchy. This involves identifying a specific fear or worry and then ranking related situations from least to most anxiety-provoking.

For example, let's say your child is afraid of dogs. Their fear ladder might look something like this:

1. Looking at pictures of friendly dogs in a book

2. Watching videos of calm dogs being petted

3. Seeing a dog on a leash from across the street

4. Standing next to a dog while a trusted adult holds the leash

5. Petting a small, gentle dog with supervision

6. Walking a friendly dog on a leash with an adult present

7. Visiting a home with a dog and interacting with it calmly

Once you have your fear ladder, the next step is to translate each level into a playful exposure activity. This is where you can get creative and tailor the play to your child's specific interests and worries.

For the child afraid of dogs, you might start by reading a silly storybook about a friendly puppy who loves to play fetch and give kisses. You could then set up a pretend veterinarian clinic, where your child gets to be the caring doctor tending to stuffed animal dogs. As they build confidence, you might watch videos together of real dogs doing cute tricks or take a walk to the park and observe dogs from a distance.

The key is to start at the bottom of the ladder, with the least challenging play scenario, and work your way up at a pace that feels manageable for your child. Please encourage them to engage with each level repeatedly until their anxiety starts to subside and they feel ready to take the next small step. And be sure to celebrate each milestone along the way, emphasizing their bravery and resilience in facing their fears.

Some other examples of translating fear ladders into playful exposures:

For a child afraid of the dark:

1. Playing with shadows and flashlights in a dimly lit room

2. Having a "glow stick dance party" with the lights off

3. Going on a pretend "midnight adventure" with a trusted stuffed animal

4. Stargazing in the backyard at dusk

5. Camping out in a blanket fort with a nightlight

6. Sleeping in their room with the door cracked open

7. Sleeping independently with the lights off

For a child afraid of public speaking:

1. Giving a mock presentation to a row of stuffed animals

2. Recording themselves telling a favorite joke or story

3. Doing a "news report" on a family member's day

4. Participating in a small group activity or game

5. Sharing a show-and-tell item with their class

6. Performing in a school play or talent show

7. Giving a speech at a family event or ceremony

As you engage in these playful exposures with your child, remember to take it slow and follow their lead. If a particular step feels too overwhelming, break it down into even smaller chunks or take a step back to a more manageable level. Be sure to model your calm and confidence throughout the process, offering reassurance and validation for your child's efforts.

With repeated practice and gentle encouragement, these gradual exposure plays can help your child rewrite their internal script around their fears. Instead of avoiding or dreading the feared situation, they can start to approach it with curiosity, courage, and even excitement. By facing their worries one playful step at a time, they can develop a deep sense of self-trust and resilience that will serve them well throughout their lives.

COMBINING RELAXATION TECHNIQUES WITH IMAGINAL EXPOSURE

While gradual exposure to play is a powerful tool for helping children face their fears, they can sometimes feel overwhelmed or triggered in the moment. That's why it's important to pair exposure with relaxation techniques that can help soothe the nervous system and promote a sense of calm and safety.

One particularly effective approach is to combine imaginal exposure – that is, facing the feared situation in one's imagination – with grounding and relaxation strategies. By coaching your child to vividly imagine their worries while simultaneously engaging in calming activities, you can help them learn that they can handle anxiety-provoking thoughts and sensations and even transform them into something more manageable.

Here's how you might guide your child through an imaginal exposure play for a specific fear or worry:

1. Set the scene: Invite your child to get comfortable in a quiet, calming space. You might dim the lights, play soft music, or even build a cozy blanket fort together. Please encourage them to bring a favorite stuffed animal or comfort object to hold during the exercise.

2. Introduce the worry: Ask your child to identify a specific fear or worry they'd like to work on. It might be something concrete, like a feared animal or situation, or something more abstract, like a worry about the future or a social interaction.

3. Guide the visualization: Invite your child to close their eyes and imagine themselves in a scenario related to their worry. Encourage them to engage all of their senses - what do they see, hear, feel, smell? Use vivid, descriptive language to help them fully immerse themselves in the imaginal scene.

4. Coach relaxation techniques: As your child engages with the imaginal exposure, guide them to simultaneously practice relaxation strategies. This might include:

- Deep belly breathing: Encourage them to take slow, deep breaths into their belly, imagining a balloon gently inflating and deflating with each inhale and exhale.
- Progressive muscle relaxation: Start at their toes and move up to their head. Have them tense, and then release each muscle group, noticing the contrast between tension and relaxation.
- Positive self-talk: Coach them to silently repeat a calming phrase or mantra, such as "I am safe," "I can handle this," or "This feeling will pass."
- Sensory grounding: Have them focus on the physical sensations of their comfort object, the soothing sound of the music, or the gentle touch of their own hands on their body.

5. Provide a soothing narrative: As your child faces their worry in their imagination, offer a gentle, reassuring narrative that emphasizes their safety and capability. You might say something like:

- "As you imagine that big, scary dog, notice how you're breathing calmly and deeply. You're in a safe space, and you have the power to control your mind and body."
- "It's okay to feel worried about that test, and at the same time, you can remember all the ways you've prepared and practiced. You have everything you need to handle this challenge, one step at a time."

6. Debrief and celebrate: After the imaginal exposure play, take a moment to debrief with your child. Ask them how it felt to face their worry in their imagination and what relaxation strategies seemed to help the most. Celebrate their courage and effort, and remind them that each time they practice this, they're building their resilience and inner strength.

With regular practice, these imaginal exposure plays can help your child develop a more flexible and adaptive response to their worries. By learning to face their fears in a safe, controlled way while simultaneously calming their mind and body, they can start to transform their relationship with anxiety from one of avoidance and dread to one of acceptance and even confidence.

Some other playful relaxation strategies you might weave into your imaginal exposure plays:

- Worry "shrinking" or "floating away": Have your child imagine their worries physically shrinking down to a tiny size or gently floating away like a balloon or a leaf on a stream.
- Power poses: Encourage your child to stand or sit in a confident, expansive posture, with their head held high and their shoulders back. This can help boost feelings of self-efficacy and courage.
- Guided imagery: Take your child on a soothing mental "vacation" to a peaceful, happy place, such as a beach, a forest, or a cozy room. Engage all of their senses to make the experience vivid and immersive.
- Art or music creation: Have your child draw, paint, or craft a representation of their worry and then transform it into something more manageable or even beautiful. Or have them compose a silly song or rhyme about their fear, focusing on their strengths and resources.

As you explore these imaginal exposure and relaxation plays with your child, remember to approach the process with lightness, creativity, and even a dash of humor. The more you can infuse the experience with a spirit of adventure and discovery, the more engaging and effective it will be.

Trust that by guiding your child to face their fears in a playful, supported way, you're giving them a priceless gift: the knowledge that they have the inner resources to handle life's challenges with grace, resilience, and even joy. You're empowering them to be the brave hero of their own story – one worry-shrinking, belly-breathing, power-posing play session at a time.

So go forth and invite your child into the wonderful world of imaginal exposures and calming play! With each gentle visualization, each soothing breath, and each triumphant grin, you're nurturing their natural capacity for courage, confidence, and inner peace. And what greater superpower could any parent hope to foster in their child than that?

EXERCISE 1: WORRY SHRINKING MACHINE

Objective:

This activity helps children visualize the process of gradually reducing the size and intensity of their worries through concrete, playful actions.

Materials:

- Cardboard boxes of various sizes (from large to small)
- Markers, stickers, or other decorating materials
- Scissors
- Worry cards or slips of paper

Instructions:

1. Introduce the concept of the Worry Shrinking Machine as a special device that can help make worries feel smaller and more manageable. Explain that the machine works by breaking down big worries into smaller, more specific parts and then applying coping strategies to shrink them down.

2. Together with the child, decorate and assemble the cardboard boxes to create the Worry Shrinking Machine. Line up the boxes from largest to smallest, and label each one with a different coping strategy (e.g., deep breathing, positive self-talk, asking for help, using humor).

3. Have the child write or draw their worries on separate cards or slips of paper. Encourage them to be specific and detailed in their descriptions.

4. Starting with the largest box, have the child place one of their worry cards inside. Ask them to describe how big and intense the worry feels on a scale of 1-10.

5. Move the worry card to the next smaller box, labeled with a coping strategy. Have the child practice that strategy for a minute or two, imagining the worry shrinking down as they do so.

6. After applying the coping strategy, have the child reassess the size and intensity of the worry. If it still feels big, repeat the process with another coping strategy in the next box.

7. Continue moving the worry card through the progressively smaller boxes, practicing a different coping strategy at each level. Encourage the child to notice how the worry feels smaller and more manageable with each step.

8. When the worry card reaches the smallest box, celebrate the child's success in shrinking it down. Have them tear up the card or throw it away, symbolizing their power over the worry.

9. Repeat the process with additional worry cards as needed, reinforcing the idea that worries can be broken down and coped with one step at a time.

Tips:

- Modify the size and number of boxes based on the child's age and attention span. For younger children, use fewer, larger boxes and simpler coping strategies.

- Allow the child to decorate and personalize the Worry Shrinking Machine to increase their sense of ownership and investment in the process.
- Model using the machine yourself with a worry of your own, verbalizing your thoughts and feelings at each step to normalize the process.

EXERCISE 2: BRAVERY BUDDY ADVENTURE

Objective:

This activity helps children practice gradual exposure to feared situations with the support and companionship of a trusted stuffed animal.

Materials:

- A stuffed animal or soft toy to serve as the child's "Bravery Buddy"
- List of feared situations or objects, ranked from least to most scary
- Calming tools or props (e.g., deep breathing card, fidget toy, positive affirmation stickers)

Instructions:

1. Introduce the concept of the Bravery Buddy as a special companion who will help the child face their fears one step at a time. Explain that Bravery Buddy has special powers of courage and calmness that the child can borrow whenever they need it.

2. Have the child choose a stuffed animal or soft toy to be their Bravery Buddy. Encourage them to give the buddy a name and backstory that highlights their brave and supportive qualities.

3. Work with the child to create a ranked list of their feared situations or objects, from least to most scary. Break down each fear into small, manageable steps that the child can practice with their Bravery Buddy.

4. Starting with the least scary situation, have the child and their Bravery Buddy approach the fear together. Encourage the child to narrate what they are experiencing and to use calming tools as needed (e.g., "My heart is beating fast, so I'm going to take some deep breaths with my buddy").

5. After completing each exposure step, have the child and their buddy celebrate their bravery with a special handshake, dance, or affirmation. Emphasize that facing fears is a process and that every small step counts.

6. As the child gains confidence with each exposure, gradually move up the list to more challenging situations. Encourage the child to lean on their Bravery Buddy for support and to imagine the buddy's courage flowing into them.

7. If the child becomes overwhelmed at any point, have them take a break with their Bravery Buddy to practice calming strategies and regroup. Emphasize that it's okay to go at their own pace and to prioritize self-care.

8. After completing the Bravery Buddy Adventure, debrief with the child about their experience. What did they learn about their bravery and resilience? How did their Bravery Buddy help them cope with their fears? What strategies do they want to remember for future challenges?

Tips:

- Personalize the Bravery Buddy to the child's specific fears and coping styles. For example, if the child fears darkness, the buddy might have a small flashlight attached, or if the child struggles with separation anxiety, the buddy might have a special goodbye ritual.
- Create a visual chart or map of the fear hierarchy to help the child track their progress and celebrate each milestone. Use stickers or markers to indicate which steps have been completed with the Bravery Buddy.
- Encourage the child to practice self-compassion and positive self-talk throughout the exposure process, just as they would support and encourage their Bravery Buddy. Model this kind and patient attitude in your language and actions.

EXERCISE 3: SUPERHERO EXPOSURE TRAINING

Objective:

This activity helps children reframe exposure to feared situations as a heroic training process, building confidence and a sense of mastery.

Materials:

- Superhero costumes or props (e.g., capes, masks, shields)
- List of feared situations or objects, ranked from least to most challenging
- Superhero-themed rewards or badges for each level of exposure

Instructions:

1. Introduce the concept of Superhero Exposure Training as a special program designed to help brave heroes like the child build their courage and face their fears. Explain that all superheroes start with small challenges and work their way up to bigger ones, just like the child will do in this activity.

2. Have the child choose a superhero persona and costume that makes them feel brave and powerful. Encourage them to create a superhero name and backstory that highlights their unique strengths and abilities.

3. Work with the child to create a ranked list of their feared situations or objects, from least to most challenging. Frame each level as a specific "mission" or "challenge" that the child will need to complete in their superhero training.

4. Starting with the least challenging mission, have the child suit up in their superhero gear and approach the situation with confidence. Encourage them to use their superhero powers (i.e., coping strategies) to manage any anxiety or discomfort that arises.

5. After completing each mission, have the child celebrate their success with a superhero pose, catchphrase, or victory dance. Present them with a special badge or reward that signifies their achievement and progress in the training program.

6. As the child gains confidence with each exposure, gradually move up the list to more challenging missions.

Encourage them to draw on their superhero strengths and to remember their past successes when facing new fears.

7. If the child becomes overwhelmed at any point, have them take a superhero "power break" to recharge their courage and practice their coping strategies. Emphasize that even superheroes need to take care of themselves and ask for help when needed.

8. After completing the Superhero Exposure Training, debrief with the child about their experience. What did they learn about their bravery and resilience? How did their superhero persona help them face their fears? What strategies do they want to keep using in their everyday life?

Tips:

- Tailor the superhero theme to the child's interests and preferences. Some children may prefer a specific comic book hero, while others may want to create their unique character.
- Use visual aids or props to make the exposure training feel more immersive and engaging. For example, create a superhero "control center" where the child can track their progress and receive their mission briefings.
- Incorporate fantasy and imagination into the exposure process to help the child distance themselves from the fear and approach it with a sense of play. For example, have them imagine shooting "courage lasers" or activating a "bravery force field" when facing a challenging situation.

EXERCISE 4: WORRY WALL TEAR-DOWN

Objective:

This activity helps children externalize and physically confront their worries, using a playful demolition metaphor to symbolize their power to overcome fears.

Materials:

- Cardboard boxes or plastic building blocks
- Paper and markers
- Soft foam balls or beanbags labeled with coping strategies
- Safety goggles or protective gear (optional)

Instructions:

1. Introduce the concept of the Worry Wall as a physical representation of the child's fears and anxieties. Explain that sometimes worries can feel like big, solid obstacles in our way but that we have the power to break them down and overcome them.

2. Have the child write or draw their specific worries on separate pieces of paper. Encourage them to be detailed and honest in their descriptions while also validating their feelings and experiences.

3. Work with the child to build a "Worry Wall" out of cardboard boxes or plastic blocks, stacking them securely but not too densely. Attach the worry papers to the front of the wall, creating a visual representation of the child's fears.

4. Have the child stand back and observe the Worry Wall, noticing any physical sensations or emotions that arise. Validate their feelings and emphasize that it's normal to feel intimidated or overwhelmed by our worries sometimes.

5. Introduce the "Coping Strategy Balls" as special tools that can help the child break through the Worry Wall. Have them !abel each ball with a different coping strategy, such as deep breathing, positive self-talk, visualization, or asking for help.

6. Have the child put on their safety gear (if using) and get ready to tear down the Worry Wall. Encourage them to choose a Coping Strategy Ball and say the corresponding strategy aloud before throwing it at the wall.

7. As the child throws each ball, have them imagine the coping strategy weakening and breaking down the worry it hits. Encourage them to use positive self-talk and affirmations as they demolish the wall (e.g., "I am stronger than my fears," "I can handle this one step at a time").

8. Once the Worry Wall is completely torn down, have the child celebrate their success with a victory cheer or dance. Emphasize that they have the power and tools to confront and overcome their fears, even if it takes time and practice.

9. Debrief with the child about their experience. What did it feel like to see their worries externalized in the wall? How did it feel to actively break them down with coping strategies? What strategies do they want to keep using in their daily life?

Tips:

- Adapt the materials and demolition process to the child's age and physical abilities. For younger children, use soft foam blocks and balls and have them knock down the wall by hand. For older children, consider using a Nerf gun or water balloons for added excitement.
- Have the child decorate the Coping Strategy Balls to make them more personalized and meaningful. Encourage them to use colors, symbols, or images that remind them of strength and resilience.
- Take photos or videos of the Worry Wall Tear-Down to create a visual reminder of the child's bravery and progress. Review these images with the child when they are feeling overwhelmed by future worries or fears.

EXERCISE 5: WHAT'S THE WORST THAT COULD HAPPEN?

Objective:

This activity helps children confront their catastrophic thinking and gain perspective on their fears by imagining worst-case scenarios in a playful, exaggerated way.

Materials:

- Paper and pencils/markers
- Silly props or costumes (optional)

Instructions:

1. Introduce the concept of catastrophic thinking as the tendency to jump to the worst possible outcome in a

feared situation. Explain that while it's normal to have these kinds of thoughts sometimes, they can often make our fears feel bigger and more unmanageable than they really are.

2. Have the child choose a specific fear or worry that they tend to catastrophize about. Ask them to describe their typical worst-case scenario for this situation, encouraging them to be as detailed and imaginative as possible.

3. Together, brainstorm a list of even more exaggerated, silly, or absurd worst-case scenarios for the same situation. Encourage the child to think of the most ridiculous and far-fetched outcomes they can imagine, such as "I'll forget my lines in the school play, and the audience will throw tomatoes at me" or "I'll fail my math test and have to live under a bridge and eat bugs for the rest of my life."

4. Have the child choose one of the silliest worst-case scenarios and act it out together, using props, costumes, or exaggerated body language to bring the scene to life. Encourage them to give it up and embrace the absurdity of the situation.

5. After acting out the scenario, have the child rate how likely they think this outcome actually is on a scale of 1-10. Discuss the difference between their catastrophic thoughts and the realistic probability of the worst-case happening.

6. Next, have the child brainstorm a list of more likely, manageable outcomes for the same situation. Encourage them to think of neutral or even positive possibilities, such as "I might stumble over a few lines in the play, but I'll keep going, and the audience will still clap" or "I might not do well on this math test, but I can ask for help and study harder for the next one."

7. Have the child act out one of the more realistic scenarios, using a calm and confident demeanor. Encourage them to notice the difference in their body sensations and emotions when imagining a manageable outcome versus a catastrophic one.

8. Debrief with the child about their experience. What did they notice about the impact of their catastrophic thinking on their fear level? How did it feel to imagine and act out more realistic or positive outcomes? What perspective shifts do they want to remember for future worries?

Tips:

- Use humor and playfulness throughout the activity to help the child gain distance from their fears and approach them with a lighter touch. Encourage silly voices, exaggerated movements, and laughter whenever possible.
- Model the process of generating and acting out worst-case scenarios yourself, using your worries or fears as examples. Emphasize that everyone has catastrophic thoughts sometimes and that they don't have to be taken seriously.
- Encourage the child to practice this technique on their own whenever they notice themselves catastrophizing. Have them keep a journal or sketchbook of their silly worst-case scenarios and realistic alternatives to look back on for perspective.

By engaging in these playful exposure and cognitive restructuring activities, children can learn to approach their worries and fears with greater flexibility, resilience, and self-compassion. Through gradual challenges, coping skill rehearsal, and humor, they can build a sense of mastery and perspective that will serve them well in navigating life's uncertainties. Remember to celebrate each small victory along the way and model a brave, playful approach to facing fears in your own life.

CHAPTER 12: BUILDING EMOTIONAL REGULATION SKILLS ONE GAME AT A TIME

PLAYING GAMES THAT PRACTICE IMPULSE CONTROL AND FLEXIBLE THINKING

Imagine you're at a birthday party, and the host announces that it's time for a game of "Red Light, Green Light." You line up with the other guests at one end of the yard, quivering with anticipation. The host shouts, "Green light!" and you dash forward with glee, feeling the wind in your hair and the grass beneath your feet. Suddenly, the host yells, "Red light!" and you must freeze in place, resisting every impulse to keep running or even twitch a muscle. The moment seems to stretch on forever until, finally, you hear "Green light!" and you're off again, sprinting towards the finish line with a mixture of determination and delight.

What may seem like a simple childhood game is actually a powerful exercise in emotional regulation – the ability to manage one's impulses, thoughts, and behaviors in service of a goal. When children practice skills like self-control, flexible thinking, and frustration tolerance in the context of play, they're building the neural pathways and emotional muscles they need to navigate life's challenges with greater resilience and adaptability.

One of the most effective ways to help children develop these regulation skills is through games that target specific cognitive and behavioral capacities. By providing clear rules, engaging challenges, and built-in opportunities for coaching and praise, these games create a safe, fun environment for children to practice regulating their emotions and actions.

Here are some classic games that can be adapted to different developmental levels and used as skill-building drills:

1. "Red Light, Green Light" for self-control: As described above, this game challenges children to start and stop their movements in response to external cues. By practicing inhibiting their impulses and delaying gratification, they're strengthening their ability to control their behavior in service of a goal.

2. "Simon Says" for inhibitory control: In this game, players must follow the leader's commands, but only when preceded by the phrase "Simon says." This requires children to pay close attention, discriminate between relevant and irrelevant cues, and inhibit the automatic response to follow every command.

3. "Freeze Dance" for self-monitoring: In this variation on musical chairs, children dance freely while the music plays but must freeze in place as soon as it stops. This game encourages children to monitor their behavior, quickly shift gears, and regulate their bodies in response to changing stimuli.

4. "Guess My Rule" for cognitive flexibility: In this game, the leader secretly chooses a rule that determines which objects or actions are allowed (e.g., only red toys or only clapping hands). Players must guess the rule by testing different hypotheses and adjusting their behavior based on feedback. This game challenges children to think flexibly, consider multiple possibilities, and adapt their strategies in response to new information.

5. "Jenga" or "Topple Tower" for frustration tolerance: In these stacking games, players take turns removing blocks from a tower and placing them on top, trying to keep the structure standing as long as possible. As the tower grows increasingly unstable, children must manage their anxiety, take calculated risks, and cope with the disappointment of an inevitable collapse.

As children engage in these games, parents can provide coaching and reinforcement to help them build and generalize their regulation skills. This might sound like:

- "I see you really want to keep running, but you're doing a great job staying still and waiting for the green light. That takes a lot of self-control!"
- "Oops, she didn't say 'Simon says,' but you followed the command anyway. That's okay – it's tricky to stop yourself sometimes! Let's see if you can catch it next time."
- "You look frustrated that the tower fell on your turn. It's so hard when that happens! Take a deep breath, and let's see if we can build it even taller this time."
- "I noticed you tried a few different rules before you figured out the pattern. Great job being flexible and keeping at it even when your first guesses didn't work out!"

By providing specific, process-oriented praise, parents can help children internalize a sense of themselves as capable, resilient learners who can handle challenges and setbacks. By joining in the play with enthusiasm and empathy, parents can model their emotional regulation skills and create a safe, supportive environment for children to practice and grow.

Of course, games are just one tool in the emotional regulation toolbox. In the next section, we'll explore how art and sensory play can help children build awareness of their internal experiences, express their feelings in healthy ways, and discover soothing strategies that work for their unique sensory needs and preferences.

USING ART AND SENSORY PLAY TO EXPLORE FEELINGS AND CALM DOWN

Imagine you're feeling overwhelmed by a swirl of big, confusing emotions. Your heart is racing, your mind is spinning, and you don't quite have the words to express what's going on inside. Now imagine that someone hands you a piece of paper and some colorful markers and invites you to draw what your feelings look like. As you begin to swirl the colors around the page, creating jagged lines or soft, blurry shapes, you start to feel a sense of release and clarity. The abstract images help you externalize and make sense of your internal experience, while the repetitive motions and sensory input help soothe your overactive nervous system.

This is the power of art and sensory play for emotional regulation—it provides a nonverbal, experiential way for children to explore, express, and manage their feelings. By engaging multiple senses and using symbolic representation, these creative activities bypass the limitations of language and logic, allowing children to process their emotions in a more intuitive, embodied way.

Here are some ideas for using art and sensory play to build emotional awareness and self-soothing skills:

1. Feelings Color Wheel: Provide your child with a paper plate or cardboard circle and invite them to divide it into wedges, like a pie chart or color wheel. Ask them to choose a color to represent each basic emotion (e.g., red for anger, blue for sadness, yellow for happiness) and fill in the wedges accordingly. Please encourage them to use the colors to show how they're feeling throughout the day or to identify the emotions of characters in stories or real-life situations.

2. *Feelings Forecast:* Invite your child to create a "weather report" for their internal emotional state, using art supplies to represent different feelings. They might use cotton balls for "cloudy" confusion, red streaks for "lightning" anger, or blue drops for "rainy" sadness. Please encourage them to notice how their emotional weather shifts throughout the day and to experiment with different art techniques to capture those changes.

3. *Calm-Down Collage:* Provide your child with a variety of soothing tactile materials, such as felt, cotton balls, feathers, and silk. Invite them to create a collage that represents calmness and safety, gluing the materials onto a piece of cardboard or paper. Please encourage them to touch and feel the different textures as they work, noticing how each one impacts their body and mind. Display the finished collage in a prominent place, and invite your child to visit it whenever they need a moment of grounding and self-soothing.

4. *Feelings Faces Playdough:* Provide your child with playdough in a variety of colors and invite them to create faces that represent different emotions. They might shape the dough into wide-open mouths or furrowed brows for anger, drooping eyelids or downturned lips for sadness, or bright, round cheeks for happiness. As they shape and mold the playdough, encourage them to notice how their facial muscles and body posture shift to match the emotion they're representing.

5. *Calming Glitter Jar:* Help your child create their own "mind jar" or "glitter bottle" by filling a clear plastic jar or bottle with water, adding a generous amount of glitter glue or liquid watercolor, and sealing the lid tightly. Invite them to shake the jar vigorously, noticing how the glitter swirls and churns like their own racing thoughts or big feelings. Then, have them set the jar down and watch as the glitter gradually settles to the bottom, imagining their mind and body becoming calm and still.

As children engage in these art and sensory activities, parents can provide gentle guidance and reflection to help them build emotional awareness and regulation skills. This might sound like:

- "I noticed you used a lot of red and orange in your feelings wheel today. What do those colors mean to you? What might have triggered those big feelings?"
- "As you're molding that playdough face, notice how your face and body feel. Are your muscles tight or relaxed? Is your breath fast or slow? What could you do to help your body feel calm and safe?"
- "Watching that glitter settle is so soothing. It reminds me that even when our feelings are really big and swirly, they will eventually pass. We can ride out the storm and find our way back to calm."

By providing a safe, nonjudgmental space for children to explore their emotions through art and sensory play, parents can help them develop a greater sense of self-awareness, self-acceptance, and self-regulation. By joining in the creative process with curiosity and empathy, parents can model their healthy ways of experiencing and expressing emotions.

It's important to note that these activities are not about creating perfect or aesthetically pleasing products but rather about the process of emotional exploration and expression. Please encourage your child to focus on the sensations, rhythms, and symbolic representations that feel meaningful to them rather than worrying about the result.

Over time, as children internalize these creative coping strategies, they may start to naturally gravitate towards art and sensory play as a way to regulate their emotions and self-soothe in challenging moments. They may also start to develop their unique variations and preferences, such as humming a certain tune when they're anxious or doodling specific patterns when they're sad.

By providing a variety of art and sensory materials and encouraging open-ended, child-led exploration, parents can support their children in developing a flexible, adaptive toolkit for emotional regulation. By creating a family culture that values creative expression and emotional honesty, parents can foster a sense of safety, connection, and resilience that will serve their children well throughout their lives.

So go ahead—break out the finger paints, playdough, and glitter glue, and dive into the messy, colorful world of emotional art and sensory play! With each squish of the clay, stroke of the brush, and swirl of the glitter jar, you're helping your child build the skills and confidence they need to navigate life's ups and downs with creativity, courage, and compassion. And what could be more beautiful than that?

EXERCISE 1: EMOTION VOLCANO FREEZE DANCE

Objective:

This activity helps children practice regulating their energy levels and emotions through physical movement and controlled breathing.

Materials:

- Music player with fast and slow songs
- Space to move and dance
- Optional: Volcano props or decorations

Instructions:

1. Introduce the concept of an Emotion Volcano as a metaphor for how our feelings can sometimes build up and overflow, like lava from a volcano. Explain that when we feel our emotions getting too big or intense, we can use strategies like movement and breathing to help regulate them.

2. Set up the play area with volcano-themed decorations, such as red and orange streamers, paper mache rocks, or a cardboard volcano cutout. Create a designated "dance floor" space in the center.

3. Explain the rules of the Emotion Volcano Freeze Dance: When the fast "lava music" plays, the child will dance and move their body energetically, as if their emotions are bubbling up inside them. When the music suddenly stops, they must freeze in place and practice deep belly breathing until the music resumes.

4. Model the game for the child, exaggerating your fast and furious dance moves when the lava music is on, then stopping abruptly and taking slow, exaggerated breaths when it stops. Encourage the child to mirror your movements and breathing.

5. Play several rounds of the game, alternating between fast and slow songs to simulate the rise and fall of emotional energy. Encourage the child to experiment with different dance moves and breathing techniques (e.g., counting breaths, snake breaths) during the freeze periods.

6. As the game progresses, introduce variations, such as having the child suggest specific emotions to embody during the dance (e.g., anger, excitement, anxiety) or using props like scarves or ribbons to represent the flow of emotions.

7. After several rounds, have the child lie down on the floor and place their hands on their belly. Guide them through a final calming breath sequence, noticing how their body and mind feel after the volcano dance.

8. Debrief with the child about their experience. What did they notice about how their body and emotions shifted throughout the game? What breathing techniques or movements felt most helpful for regulating their energy? How might they use this strategy in real-life situations when their emotions feel overwhelming?

Tips:

- Adapt the game to the child's energy levels and preferences. Some may prefer more vigorous, full-body movements, while others may feel more comfortable with smaller, repetitive motions.
- Encourage the child to suggest their own music choices or create a themed playlist together. Consider using instrumental tracks or nature sounds for the freeze periods to facilitate relaxation.
- Incorporate visualization into the breathing practices, such as imagining the breath as a cool, calming waterfall or a gentle ocean wave washing away the hot lava of emotions.

EXERCISE 2: FRUSTRATION JENGA

Objective:

This activity helps children practice problem-solving and coping with frustrating situations through a playful, cooperative twist on a classic game.

Materials:

- Jenga set
- Markers or stickers
- List of age-appropriate frustrating situations

Instructions:

1. Before playing, write or print out a list of common frustrating situations that the child might encounter, such as "You can't find your favorite toy," "Your sibling won't share the iPad," or "You're stuck on a difficult homework problem."

2. Label each Jenga block with a different frustrating situation using the markers or stickers. Try to include a variety of scenarios that cover different areas of the child's life (e.g., school, home, friends).

3. Set up the Jenga tower according to the standard rules, but explain that this game will have a special twist: Each time a player successfully removes a block, they must read aloud the frustrating situation written on it.

4. The player then shares one idea for how they could cope with or solve that particular situation. Encourage them to think of strategies that are realistic, helpful, and kind to themselves and others.

5. The other players can offer additional suggestions or support, but the focus should be on the active players generating their solutions. Validate their ideas and encourage creative thinking.

6. If the player gets stuck or frustrated, model coping strategies such as taking deep breaths, asking for help, or breaking the problem down into smaller steps. Emphasize that it's okay to feel frustrated sometimes and that

there are always ways to work through it.

7. Continue playing the game as usual, with each player taking turns removing blocks and sharing coping ideas for the frustrating situations. If the tower falls, work together to rebuild it and keep practicing problem-solving.

8. After the game, debrief with the child about their experience. What coping strategies did they find most helpful or interesting? How did it feel to talk through frustrating situations with others' support? What situations do they want to keep practicing problem-solving for?

Tips:

- Adapt the frustrating situations to the child's specific challenges and developmental level. For younger children, use simpler, more concrete scenarios and coping strategies.
- Encourage the child to come up with their frustrating situations to add to the game based on their real-life experiences. This can help them feel more ownership over the problem-solving process.
- Model positive self-talk and growth mindset throughout the game, such as "This is a tough situation, but I know I can find a way through it" or "Mistakes and frustrations are just opportunities to learn and grow."

EXERCISE 3: HEART AND MIND HOPSCOTCH

Objective:

This activity helps children explore the connection between thoughts and emotions through a playful, physical game that combines hopscotch with cognitive reframing.

Materials:

- Sidewalk chalk or masking tape
- Small throwable object (e.g., beanbag, stone)
- Emotion and thought cards (optional)

Instructions:

1. Using the chalk or tape, create a hopscotch board on the ground with 8-10 squares. In each square, draw a different emotion face (e.g., happy, sad, angry, scared, excited, proud).

2. Explain the rules of Heart and Mind Hopscotch: The child will throw the small object onto the board, then hop to that square, avoiding the square with the object. When they land on the emotion face, they must say aloud a thought that someone might have if they were feeling that way.

3. Model the game for the child, exaggerating the emotional expressions as you land on each face. Share a corresponding thought, such as "I'm having so much fun!" for the happy face or "I'll never be able to do this" for the sad face.

4. Have the child take a turn throwing the object and hopping to the square. Encourage them to really get into character as they make the emotional face and share a related thought. Validate their responses and offer praise for their efforts.

5. As the game progresses, introduce the idea of reframing negative thoughts into more helpful or accurate ones.

For example, if the child lands on the angry face and says, "It's not fair, I never get to choose the game," you could suggest a reframe like, "I'm frustrated right now, but I know we can take turns choosing the game."

6. Encourage the child to generate their own reframes for the negative thoughts, focusing on perspective-taking, problem-solving, and self-compassion. Offer guidance and support as needed, but let them take the lead in finding alternative ways of thinking.

7. Play several rounds of the game, taking turns hopping and sharing thoughts and reframes. Notice any patterns or themes that emerge in the child's responses and reflect them with curiosity and empathy.

8. After the game, debrief with the child about their experience. What did they notice about the relationship between their thoughts and emotions? How did it feel to reframe negative thoughts into more helpful ones? What strategies do they want to remember for managing difficult emotions in real life?

Tips:

- Adapt the game to the child's developmental level by adjusting the complexity of the emotions and thoughts. For younger children, use simpler, more concrete feeling words and visual supports like pictures or stickers.
- Encourage the child to come up with their emotional faces and corresponding thoughts to add to the game. They could even create their hopscotch board with personalized themes or challenges.
- Extend the game by having the child act out a brief scenario or dialogue based on the emotion, face, and thought they land on. This can help them practice embodying and expressing different feeling states in a playful, low-stakes way.

EXERCISE 4: CALM DOWN CORNERS

Objective:

This activity helps children practice identifying and using different coping strategies for emotional regulation through a multi-sensory, interactive game.

Materials:

- Designated play area with 4-5 different "calm down corners"
- Each corner should have a specific theme and corresponding materials, such as:
- Breathing corner: Pinwheels, bubbles, feathers, guided breathing cards
- Movement corner: Yoga mats, stretchy bands, balance cushions, dance ribbons
- Sensory corner: Fidget toys, stress balls, kinetic sand, calming scents or lotions
- Art corner: Coloring pages, markers, paints, playdough, calming music
- Relaxation corner: Soft blankets or pillows, stuffed animals, calming books or audio stories

Instructions:

1. Before playing, set up the designated play area with 4-5 different "calm down corners," each with a specific theme and corresponding materials. Arrange the materials in an inviting, accessible way that encourages exploration and engagement.

2. Introduce the concept of Calm Down Corners as special places to visit when big emotions arise, each with its own set of tools and strategies for feeling better. Explain that different people find different things helpful for calming down and that it's important to have a variety of options to choose from.

3. Give the child a brief tour of each corner, modeling how to use the different materials and explaining how each strategy can help with emotional regulation. Encourage the child to explore the corners on their own and notice which ones feel most appealing or helpful to them.

4. Play a game where you take turns spinning a spinner or drawing cards with different emotion words (e.g., angry, sad, worried, frustrated). When an emotion is selected, the child must go to one of the Calm Down Corners and choose a tool or strategy to practice for a few minutes as if they were feeling that way.

5. As the child engages with each corner, ask them to notice how their body and mind feel before, during, and after using the coping strategy. Encourage them to rate their distress level on a scale of 1-10 and observe any changes.

6. After practicing in each corner, have the child reflect on their experience. Which strategies did they find most enjoyable or effective? How did it feel to have a variety of options to choose from? What corners would they want to visit in real life when big emotions arise?

7. Brainstorm with the child how they can create their own Calm Down Corner at home or in the classroom with personalized tools and strategies that work best for them. Make a plan to gather the necessary materials and set up the space together.

8. Encourage the child to visit their Calm Down Corner regularly, both when they are feeling dysregulated and when they are calm, to build comfort and mastery of the different coping strategies. Model using the space yourself and share your own experiences with emotional regulation.

Tips:

- Adapt the corners to the child's sensory preferences and developmental needs. Some children may prefer more active, movement-based strategies, while others may gravitate towards quieter, sensory-based activities.
- Rotate the materials in each corner periodically to maintain novelty and engagement. Consider seasonal themes or integrating the child's favorite characters or interests.
- Create a visual menu or choice board of the different coping strategies to help the child remember their options in the moment of dysregulation. Use pictures, symbols, or keywords to represent each corner or tool.
- Encourage the child to reflect on their Calm Down Corner experiences in a journal or through art. This can help them process their emotions and internalize the coping strategies over time.

EXERCISE 5: FEELINGS FINGERPAINTING

Objective:

This activity helps children explore and express their emotions through a sensory-rich, creative process that encourages self-awareness and regulation.

Materials:

- Washable finger paints in a variety of colors
- Large paper or poster board
- Smocks or old clothes for mess protection
- Wet wipes or sink for easy cleanup
- Music player with speaker
- Playlist of instrumental songs that evoke different feeling states

Instructions:

1. Set up the fingerpainting area with the necessary materials, including a large sheet of paper or poster board, several colors of fingerpaint, and smocks or old clothes for mess protection.

2. Introduce the concept of Feelings Fingerpainting as a special way to express and explore our emotions through color, shape, and texture. Explain that there is no right or wrong way to paint and that the goal is to let our feelings guide our artistic choices.

3. Play a brief sample of each instrumental song on the playlist, asking the child to notice how each one makes them feel in their body and mind. Encourage them to share any colors, images, or movements that come to mind as they listen.

4. Choose one song to start with and invite the child to begin fingerpainting as the music plays, focusing on expressing the feelings that arise through their art. Encourage them to experiment with different strokes, pressure, and color combinations.

5. As the child paints, ask open-ended questions about their artistic process, such as "What does that color represent for you?" or "How did you decide to make those shapes?" Validate their responses and reflect their feelings and words to them.

6. When the song ends, have the child step back and observe their painting. Ask them to title the piece based on the dominant emotion or theme they expressed. Encourage them to share any insights or surprises they noticed about their feelings through the process.

7. Repeat the process with additional songs, using a fresh sheet of paper for each one. Encourage the child to experiment with different painting techniques or color palettes to represent the different feeling states.

8. After completing several paintings, lay them out side by side and have the child reflect on the collection as a whole. What similarities or differences do they notice across the pieces? How does each painting make them feel as they look at it now? What did they learn about their emotions through this process?

9. Display the Feelings Fingerpaintings in a special place, such as on the fridge or in the child's room. Use them as a springboard for ongoing conversations about emotional awareness and expression.

Tips:

- Adapt the activity to the child's sensory needs and preferences. Some may enjoy the messy, tactile sensation of fingerpainting, while others may prefer using brushes or sponges for a less intense experience.
- Encourage the child to use their non-dominant hand or paint with their eyes closed for an added element of mindfulness and sensory exploration.
- Extend the activity by having the child create a feelings color wheel, assigning a specific color to each basic emotion and mixing them to represent more complex feeling states. Use this as a reference tool for ongoing emotional check-ins and communication.
- Incorporate movement into the painting process by having the child dance or gesture along with the music as they create. This can help them embody and integrate the feeling states more fully.

EXERCISE 6: MINDFUL MONKEY MEMORY

Objective:

This activity helps children learn and practice different mindfulness strategies through a playful, interactive memory game that encourages focus, self-awareness, and emotional regulation.

Materials:

- Memory game cards with mindfulness activity pictures, such as:
- Deep breathing
- Progressive muscle relaxation
- Mindful listening
- Body scan
- Gratitude practice
- Mindful eating
- Five senses grounding
- Visualization
- Quiet, comfortable space to play

Instructions:

1. Before playing, create or purchase a set of memory game cards with different mindfulness activity pictures. Each activity should have a matching pair of cards.

2. Shuffle the cards and lay them out face down in a grid pattern on a flat surface, such as a table or floor.

3. Introduce the concept of mindfulness as paying attention to the present moment with curiosity and kindness. Explain that mindfulness can help us feel calmer, more focused, and more in control of our emotions.

4. Demonstrate how to play Mindful Monkey Memory: Players take turns flipping over two cards at a time,

trying to find matching pairs. When a match is found, the player keeps the cards and takes another turn. The game continues until all pairs have been matched.

5. Introduce the mindfulness twist: Each time a player finds a matching pair, they must demonstrate or explain the mindfulness activity shown on the cards. The other player(s) then follow along and practice the activity together for a minute or two.

6. As each mindfulness activity is practiced, encourage the child to notice how it feels in their body and mind. Ask them to describe any sensations, thoughts, or emotions that arise using curious, non-judgmental language.

7. After completing a few rounds of the game, take a break and reflect on the different mindfulness activities experienced so far. Which ones did the child enjoy most? Which ones felt challenging or unfamiliar? What benefits did they notice from practicing mindfulness, even briefly?

8. Continue playing the game until all pairs have been matched and all mindfulness activities have been practiced. Encourage the child to take their time and really engage with each activity rather than rushing through to find the next match.

9. At the end of the game, debrief with the child about their overall experience. What did they learn about mindfulness through the different activities? How do they feel different in their body and mind compared to when they started? What activities would they like to incorporate into their daily routine?

10. Make a plan with the child to practice their favorite mindfulness activities regularly, both during calm times and in moments of stress or dysregulation. Brainstorm specific cues or reminders to help them remember to use their mindfulness skills throughout the day.

Tips:

- Adapt the mindfulness activities to the child's developmental level and attention span. For younger children, use simpler, more concrete practices like belly breathing or sensory grounding. For older children, introduce more abstract concepts like visualization or gratitude.
- Create your mindfulness memory cards with images and instructions that resonate with the child's interests and learning style. Consider using photos of the children themselves practicing each activity for a more personalized touch.
- Extend the activity by having the child teach their favorite mindfulness practices to friends or family members. This can help reinforce their understanding and build a sense of mastery and leadership.
- Incorporate mindfulness language and prompts into other games or activities, such as pausing for a mindful moment before taking a turn or using a breathing exercise as a "reset" button when frustration arises.

By engaging in these playful, experiential activities, children can develop a toolkit of emotional regulation skills that they can draw on throughout their lives. Through games like Emotion Volcano Freeze Dance, Frustration Jenga, Heart and Mind Hopscotch, Calm Down Corners, Feelings Fingerpainting, and Mindful Monkey Memory, children learn to identify, express, and manage their emotions in healthy, adaptive ways.

As a caregiver, your role is to model these skills yourself, create a safe and supportive environment for practice, and offer guidance and reinforcement along the way. Remember to approach the process with patience, creativity, and a spirit of self-compassion - both for yourself and for the child. With time and consistent practice, emotional regulation will become a natural, integrated part of the child's life, helping them navigate challenges with resilience and grace.

Part 4: Dialectical-Behavioral Play Interventions

CHAPTER 13: CULTIVATING MINDFULNESS THROUGH PLAYFUL EXERCISES

INTRODUCING MINDFULNESS CONCEPTS TO CHILDREN

In our fast-paced, constantly connected world, the practice of mindfulness has emerged as a powerful tool for promoting well-being, resilience, and emotional balance. But what exactly is mindfulness, and how can we make this abstract concept accessible and engaging for children?

At its core, mindfulness is the simple but profound act of bringing our full attention to the present moment with openness, curiosity, and acceptance. It's about tuning into our immediate experience – the sights, sounds, sensations, and feelings that are unfolding right here, right now – without getting caught up in judgments, worries, or distractions. When we practice mindfulness, we step out of the churning stream of our thoughts and into the still, clear pool of present-moment awareness.

For children, who are naturally wired to live in the moment, mindfulness is an innate capacity that can be nurtured and strengthened through playful, age-appropriate exercises. By learning to pay attention to purpose and observing their inner and outer experiences with kindness and curiosity, children can develop a powerful set of skills for navigating life's challenges with greater ease and resilience.

Some of the key benefits of mindfulness for children include:

1. Reduced stress and anxiety: By learning to anchor themselves in the present moment, children can break free from the grip of worried thoughts about the future or regrets about the past. Mindfulness helps them cultivate a sense of inner calm and stability, even in the face of external stressors.

2. Enhanced emotional regulation: Mindfulness teaches children to observe their emotions with gentle, nonjudgmental awareness rather than getting overwhelmed by them. By creating a sense of space and perspective around their feelings, children can respond to challenges with greater flexibility and skill.

3. Increased focus and attention: Mindfulness exercises help children strengthen their "attention muscle," improving their ability to concentrate, retain information, and resist distractions. These skills are crucial for success in school and beyond.

4. Greater self-awareness and self-compassion: By tuning into their thoughts, feelings, and physical sensations with curiosity and acceptance, children develop a deeper understanding of themselves and their needs. They learn to treat themselves with kindness and compassion rather than harsh self-judgment.

5. Enhanced appreciation and savoring: Mindfulness opens children up to the richness and beauty of the present moment, helping them notice and appreciate the small joys and wonders of life that might otherwise go unnoticed. This cultivation of gratitude and savoring is a key ingredient of lasting happiness.

So, how can we introduce these powerful concepts to children in a way that is engaging, concrete, and developmentally appropriate? One helpful approach is to use simple, relatable analogies and metaphors that make mindfulness come alive for kids.

For example, you might compare the mind to a busy train station, with thoughts and feelings constantly arriving and departing like trains. Mindfulness is like being the calm, friendly station master who greets each train with a warm smile but doesn't hop on board and get carried away by them.

Or you might talk about mindfulness as being like a superhero with special powers of observation and acceptance. Just like a superhero uses their x-ray vision to see beneath the surface of things, mindfulness helps us look closely at our own inner experience with clarity and curiosity. And just like a superhero stays calm and focused in the face of danger, mindfulness helps us stay grounded and balanced even when big feelings arise.

You can also introduce mindfulness concepts through playful, experiential exercises that allow children to discover the power of present-moment awareness for themselves. For example, you might guide them through a "mindful eating" exercise, where they take a single raisin or piece of chocolate and engage all of their senses to explore it fully before eating. Or you might play a "listening game," where you take turns closing your eyes and seeing how many different sounds you can notice in the environment around you.

The key is to keep the tone light, curious, and exploratory rather than didactic or prescriptive. Mindfulness is not about achieving a particular state or outcome but about cultivating a friendly, open relationship with our moment-to-moment experience, whatever it may be.

As a parent, one of the most powerful ways you can introduce mindfulness to your child is by modeling it yourself. Take opportunities throughout the day to pause, take a deep breath, and tune into your senses and surroundings. Share your observations and experiences with your child using simple, concrete language. When your child is experiencing a strong emotion or challenging situation, guide them to take a mindful pause and check in with their inner experience before reacting.

With regular practice and playful exploration, mindfulness can become a natural, integral part of your child's daily life – a source of inner strength, clarity, and joy that they can draw upon for years to come. In the next section, we'll explore some specific games and activities that you can use to help your child develop and practice these invaluable skills.

ENGAGING IN GAMES AND ACTIVITIES FOR PRACTICING MINDFULNESS SKILLS

Now that we've introduced the basic concepts of mindfulness in a kid-friendly way, let's dive into some fun, interactive games and activities that can help children practice and strengthen their mindfulness muscles. These exercises are designed to promote key mindfulness skills such as focused attention, body awareness, emotional regulation, and sensory exploration, all in a playful, engaging format that meets children where they are.

Remember, the goal of these activities is not to achieve a particular outcome or state of relaxation but to help children cultivate a friendly, curious relationship with their present-moment experience. Keep the tone light and exploratory, and be sure to model your engagement and enjoyment of the process.

Here are a few ideas to get you started:

1. Belly Buddy Breathing:

Please have your child lie down on their back and place a small stuffed animal on their belly. Encourage them to focus their attention on the sensation of the toy rising and falling with each breath, as if they are giving their "belly buddy" a gentle ride. You can make it a game by having them try to keep the toy as still as possible or see how slowly and smoothly they can make it rise and fall. This exercise helps children tune into the physical sensations of breathing and use it as an anchor for present-moment awareness.

2. Body Squeeze:

Guide your child to lie down on their back and imagine they are a tube of toothpaste. Starting at their toes, have them squeeze and tense each part of their body in turn as if they are squeezing out all the "toothpaste." Work your way up to the top of their head, then have them release all the tension and "squish" out like an empty tube. This progressive muscle relaxation exercise helps children develop body awareness, release physical tension, and practice the skill of letting go.

3. Safari Senses Scavenger Hunt:

Take your child on an imaginary "safari" around your home or yard, and have them use their senses to explore the environment like a curious animal. You might say something like, "Let's pretend we're baby deer exploring the forest for the first time. What do your deer ears hear? What does your deer nose smell? What do your deer eyes see?" Please encourage them to really tune into the small, subtle details of their sensory experience and share their observations with excitement and wonder. This exercise helps children cultivate sensory awareness, curiosity, and appreciation for the richness of the present moment.

4. Mindful Movement:

Put on some music with a strong, steady beat and guide your child to move their body in sync with the rhythm. Please encourage them to really tune into the physical sensations of each movement, noticing how it feels in their muscles, bones, and skin. You can make it a game by calling out different body parts or movement qualities for them to focus on, such as "Now let's move just our elbows!" or "Can you make your movements sharp and spiky like a porcupine?" This exercise combines body awareness, focused attention, and playful creativity.

5. Heartbeat Buddy:

Have your child choose a favorite stuffed animal or toy to be their "heartbeat buddy." Guide them to hold the toy close to their chest and focus on the sensation of their heartbeat. You can make it a game by having them count how many beats they feel in one minute or see if they can sync their breathing to the rhythm of their heart. This exercise helps children tune into their internal physical experience and practice using it as an anchor for present-moment awareness.

6. Weather Report:

Guide your child to sit or lie down comfortably, and imagine that they are a weather reporter giving a "weather report" about their inner experience. Please encourage them to tune into their physical sensations, emotions, and thoughts and describe them in weather-related terms. For example, they might say something like, "Right now, in my body, I notice a warm, tingly sun shining in my belly. In my mind, I see some scattered clouds of worry about my math test, but there's also a cool breeze of excitement about playing with my friends later." This exercise helps children develop self-awareness, emotional literacy, and the ability to observe their inner experiences with descriptive, non-judgmental language.

As you explore these and other mindfulness games with your child, be sure to adapt them to their unique interests, abilities, and developmental stages. Use language and metaphors that resonate with their experience, and follow their lead in terms of pacing and engagement. Remember to celebrate their efforts and observations with genuine enthusiasm and appreciation.

Over time, as your child internalizes these mindfulness skills through regular practice and play, you may start to notice subtle shifts in their ability to regulate their emotions, focus their attention, and savor the good things in life. They may become more adept at taking a mindful pause before reacting to challenges or more curious and accepting of their inner landscape.

But perhaps the greatest gift of these mindfulness exercises is the way they nurture your child's innate capacity for wonder, joy, and connection – both to themselves and to the world around them. By learning to tune into the magic and mystery of the present moment, your child develops a deep sense of inner peace, wholeness, and resilience that will serve them well throughout their lives.

As you share in these mindful adventures together, you may find yourself rediscovering your childlike sense of presence, playfulness, and awe. You may feel a renewed appreciation for the simple pleasures and profound depths of this one precious life. You may come to see mindfulness not as a "technique" or "intervention" but as a way of being – a path of curiosity, compassion, and connection that you and your child can walk together, one mindful step at a time.

EXERCISE 1: BELLY BUDDY BREATHING

Objective:

This activity teaches children how to use deep belly breathing to calm their bodies and focus their minds, using a playful, tactile approach.

Materials:

- Stuffed animal or small pillow for each participant
- Comfortable place to lie down

Instructions:

1. Invite your child to lie down on their back in a comfortable position, with their head supported and their arms and legs relaxed.

2. Give your child a small stuffed animal or pillow to place on their belly, just above their belly button. Encourage them to notice how the toy rises and falls with each breath.

3. Guide your child to take slow, deep breaths into their belly as if they are filling up a balloon. Encourage them to breathe in through their nose and out through their mouth, making a soft "whoosh" sound.

4. As they inhale, ask your child to notice how their belly rises and their Belly Buddy lifts. As they exhale, have them feel their belly fall and their Belly Buddy sink.

5. Challenge your child to see how slowly and gently they can breathe, keeping their Belly Buddy steady. They might imagine their breath as a gentle ocean wave or a soft breeze.

6. Continue this deep belly breathing for several minutes until your child feels calm and centered. Encourage them to notice any changes in their body, mind, or emotions.

7. After the exercise, debrief with your child about their experience. When might Belly Buddy Breathing be helpful in their daily life? How can they remember to use this tool when they need it?

Tips:

- Model the belly breathing alongside your child using your stuffed animal or pillow. Exaggerate the rise and fall of your belly to make it visible and engaging.
- Encourage your child to name their Belly Buddy and give it a personality. They might imagine that Belly Buddy is coaching them or breathing with them.
- Try Belly Buddy Breathing in different positions, such as sitting up or standing. Notice how the sensations change in each position.
- For older children, you can add a guided body scan to the belly breathing, inviting them to notice and relax each part of their body in turn.

EXERCISE 2: SAFARI SENSES SCAVENGER HUNT

Objective:

This activity promotes mindful awareness of the present moment by encouraging children to engage all of their senses in a playful, exploratory way.

Materials:

- List of sensory scavenger hunt items (see sample below)
- Bags or baskets for collecting items
- Optional: Magnifying glasses, binoculars, or other sensory aids

Instructions:

1. Introduce the Safari Senses Scavenger Hunt by inviting your child to imagine they are explorers on a safari, using all of their senses to discover the wonders of their environment.

2. Provide a list of sensory items to find on the scavenger hunt, such as:

- Something rough
- Something smooth
- Something that makes a crunching sound
- Something that smells sweet
- Something that tastes sour
- Something that looks like a circle

- Something that feels warm
- Something that sounds like music

3. Give your child a bag or basket to collect their sensory items as they find them. Encourage them to take their time and really savor each discovery, noticing as many details as possible.

4. As your child finds each item, invite them to share their observations with you. Ask open-ended questions like, "What do you notice about that leaf? How does it feel different from the bark?"

5. Challenge your child to find at least one item for each sense, but allow them to collect additional items that capture their curiosity. Encourage a spirit of appreciation and wonder.

6. After the scavenger hunt, lay out all of the collected items and invite your child to create a "sensory museum" or "mindfulness mandala" by arranging them in a meaningful way.

7. Reflect on the experience together, noticing any new insights or appreciation for the world around you. Discuss how you can bring this mindful, multisensory awareness into other parts of your day.

Tips:

- Adapt the scavenger hunt items to your child's developmental stage and your environment. For younger children, focus on simple, concrete sensations. For older children, include more abstract or nuanced prompts.
- Make the scavenger hunt a regular family ritual, such as a seasonal tradition or a vacation activity. Notice how your sensory experiences change in different settings and times of year.
- Extend the activity by creating artwork, poetry, or stories inspired by your sensory discoveries. Encourage your child to capture their mindful observations creatively.
- Use the Safari Senses framework to practice mindfulness in everyday moments, such as eating a meal, taking a walk, or doing a chore. Pause to notice and savor the sensory details of the experience.

EXERCISE 3: THOUGHT CLOUDS

Objective:

This activity teaches children how to observe their thoughts with curiosity and detachment rather than getting caught up in their content or emotional charge.

Materials:

- Comfortable place to sit or lie down
- Optional: Blue sky image or video

Instructions:

1. Invite your child to find a comfortable position, either sitting up tall or lying down on their back. Encourage them to close their eyes or soften their gaze.

2. Guide your child to take a few deep, calm breaths, noticing the sensation of the air moving in and out of their

body. Invite them to imagine they are breathing in a peaceful blue sky and breathing out any worries or tension.

3. Explain that our minds are like the sky, and our thoughts are like clouds that drift across it. Sometimes, the clouds are light and fluffy; sometimes, they are dark and stormy, but the sky is always there behind them.

4. Ask your child to begin noticing any thoughts that float into their mind without trying to change or control them. They might silently label each thought as it arises, such as "planning," "remembering," "worrying," or "imagining."

5. Encourage your child to imagine each thought gently drifting across the sky of their mind, like a cloud blown by the wind. Remind them that they don't need to hold onto the thought or follow it; they can watch it pass by.

6. If your child gets caught up in a particular thought or feeling, gently redirect their attention back to their breath and the image of the sky. Reassure them that it's natural for the mind to wander, and they can always return to observing their thoughts.

7. Continue the thought cloud observation for a few minutes or as long as your child is engaged. Invite them to notice any patterns or insights that arise during the practice.

8. After the exercise, debrief with your child about their experience. What was it like to watch their thoughts drift by? Did they notice any particular types of thought clouds? How might this practice help them handle difficult thoughts or feelings?

Tips:

- Model the thought cloud exercise alongside your child, sharing your observations and insights. Normalize the experience of having a busy or distractible mind.
- Use visual aids like pictures or videos of clouds to help your child connect with the metaphor. You might even do the exercise outdoors while watching real clouds drift by.
- Encourage your child to get creative with the thought cloud imagery, such as imagining their thoughts as leaves floating down a stream or cars driving past on a highway. The key is to cultivate a sense of detachment and movement.
- Remind your child that the goal is not to get rid of thought clouds but to change their relationship with them. They can learn to observe their thoughts with curiosity and acceptance rather than judgment or reactivity.

EXERCISE 4: SOUND OFF

Objective:

This activity cultivates mindful listening and teaches children how to use sound as an anchor for present-moment awareness.

Materials:

- Bell, chime, or singing bowl
- Quiet, comfortable space

Instructions:

1. Invite your child to find a comfortable seated position, either on a cushion or in a chair. Encourage them to sit up tall, with their shoulders relaxed and their hands resting in their lap.

2. Show your child the bell, chime, or singing bowl and demonstrate how to make a clear, resonant sound with it. Invite them to listen carefully to the sound, noticing how it begins, peaks, and fades away.

3. Explain that you will be playing a game called "Sound Off," where the goal is to listen mindfully to the sound of the bell until it completely disappears. Challenge your child to raise their hand when they can no longer hear the sound.

4. Ring the bell or chime, and invite your child to close their eyes and focus all of their attention on the sound. Encourage them to notice any physical sensations, such as vibrations in their body or ears.

5. As the sound fades, remind your child to keep listening carefully, as if they are trying to hear a whisper. When they can no longer hear the sound, even if they strain their ears, they should raise their hand.

6. Once everyone has raised their hand, take a few deep breaths together and then discuss the experience. What was it like to focus so intently on one sound? Did any other thoughts or sensations arise while they were listening?

7. Repeat the Sound Off game several times, experimenting with different lengths and volumes of sound. Encourage your child to notice how their mind and body feel before, during, and after each round.

8. After the activity, brainstorm with your child about other times when they could use mindful listening to anchor their attention and calm their mind. How might they apply this skill in daily life?

Tips:

- If you don't have a bell or chime, you can use any other resonant sound, such as a tuning fork, a guitar string, or even a glass of water that you tap with a spoon.
- Encourage your child to experiment with making the sound themselves, noticing how the vibrations feel in their hand and body. They might even try to match the length of their breath to the duration of the sound.
- Extend the activity by going on a "sound walk" together, listening mindfully to the sounds of nature or the environment around you. Take turns pointing out different sounds and describing them in detail.
- Use the Sound Off game as a quick mindfulness break throughout the day, such as before meals, before homework, or before bedtime. The simple act of listening can be a powerful way to reset and recharge.

Remember, the key to teaching mindfulness to children is to keep it playful, experiential, and relevant to their daily lives. By offering a variety of engaging activities that cultivate present-moment awareness, you help your child develop a toolkit of mindfulness skills that they can draw on for a lifetime of resilience and well-being. Enjoy exploring the magic of mindfulness together!

CHAPTER 14: FOSTERING INTERPERSONAL SKILLS THROUGH COOPERATIVE PLAY

TEACHING ASSERTIVENESS AND ACTIVE LISTENING THROUGH ROLE PLAY

Imagine your child comes home from school deflated, complaining that no one wants to play with them at recess. Or maybe they're fuming because a classmate cut in front of them in line again. Playground politics and friendship fiascos can feel like life-or-death dramas to school-aged kids who are just learning to navigate the complex world of peer relationships. As a parent, it's tempting to jump in with solutions or platitudes. But what if you could equip your child with the tools to tackle these tricky situations themselves?

Enter role-play - the ultimate dress rehearsal for real-world social challenges. By engaging your child in playful simulations of common interpersonal scenarios, you give them a safe space to experiment with different communication strategies and build confidence in their social skills. Role-playing allows kids to step into others' shoes, test out new ways of expressing themselves, and get immediate feedback on the impact of their words and actions.

One key skill that role-play can help develop is assertiveness—the ability to stand up for one's own needs and rights while respecting others. Assertive communication involves expressing feelings, opinions, and boundaries clearly, calmly, and directly without resorting to aggression or passive aggression. It's a tough balance for kids (and adults!) who may default to either people-pleasing or bullying when their needs feel threatened.

Here's an example of how you might use role play to practice assertiveness:

Scenario: Your 8-year-old is upset because a friend keeps borrowing his favorite markers without asking and not returning them.

Parent: "Okay, let's pretend I'm your friend who took your markers. Show me how you could talk to me about it."

Child: (timidly) "Um, can I have my markers back?"

Parent: "Hmm, I'm not sure which ones are yours. I need them to finish my project."

Child: (getting frustrated) "But they're mine! You can't just take them!"

Parent: "I hear how frustrated you are. Can we try that again with an 'I-statement'? Something like, 'I feel upset when you take my markers without asking. I need them too. Next time, please check with me first.'"

Child: (deep breath) "I feel mad when you keep taking my markers. I like sharing, but I need you to ask me first and give them back when you're done."

Parent: "Wow, I really understood your feelings that time. I'll be sure to ask next time. Thanks for letting me know nicely."

In this example, the parent first gives the child a chance to navigate the situation on their own. When the child struggles to express their needs effectively, the parent models an assertive I-statement and invites the child to try again. Through repetition and coaching, the child practices finding the sweet spot between the doormat and steamroller - respectfully making their case without attacking the other person.

You can use this same formula to role-play countless other scenarios:

- Asking to join a game on the playground
- Requesting a turn with a coveted toy
- Responding to teasing or exclusion
- Negotiating compromises with siblings
- Expressing hurt feelings to a friend
- Telling a grown-up about a problem

The key is to follow your child's lead in selecting scenarios that feel relevant to their world. Listen for recurring themes in their play or stories about school and friends. Notice situations that seem to trigger big feelings or challenging behaviors. Choose a few concrete examples to start with, then invite your child to come up with their variations as their skills grow.

As you role-play, coach your child to use specific assertive communication tools:

- I-statements ("I feel...when...I need...")
- Reflective listening ("What I hear you saying is...")
- Acknowledging others' perspectives ("I know you want...too.")
- Offering compromises ("How about we take turns?")
- Setting clear boundaries ("I'm not okay with that.")

It may feel awkward or stilted as you act out these exchanges, but that's part of the point! By exaggerating gestures and vocal tones, you help your child tune into the nuances of body language and verbal cues that they might miss in the heat of a real-life moment. Inject some playful humor to keep the mood light while still treating their concerns as valid and important.

Remember, the goal is not to script your child's every social move but to give them a flexible toolbox of strategies to draw from as they find their unique voice. Praise their efforts, not just their execution. Ask them how it feels to express themselves more clearly. Point out small victories as you observe them putting their new skills into practice in daily life.

With every playful rehearsal, your child is laying down new neural pathways for assertive communication and emotional intelligence. They're discovering that they have the power to advocate for themselves and connect with others in positive ways. So keep those imaginative juices flowing and watch your budding diplomat bloom!

ENHANCING COOPERATION AND TEAMWORK THROUGH GROUP GAMES

If assertiveness is about finding one's voice, cooperation is about learning to harmonize that voice with others. As kids navigate the ups and downs of friendships and sibling bonds, they quickly discover that not everyone thinks, feels, or acts the same way they do. Conflicts arise, egos clash, and feelings get hurt. But when kids learn to harness their differences and work towards common goals, magical things can happen.

Cooperative games and activities offer a fun, low-stakes way to practice collaboration, communication, and creative problem-solving skills. By tackling a shared challenge together, kids get real-time feedback on the impact of their choices and behaviors on group dynamics. They learn to listen actively, express ideas clearly, negotiate compromises, and adjust their strategies based on others' input.

One classic cooperative game is "Human Knot":

- Gather a group of 5-10 players in a circle.
- Each person reaches across and grasps the hands of two different people, creating a tangled knot of arms.
- The group must then work together to untangle themselves without breaking their hand-holds, ending up in a circle again.

This seemingly simple task requires a surprising amount of coordination, patience, and creative thinking. Players must take turns suggesting moves and guiding each other's bodies with care. They have to stay attuned to the group's progress as a whole, not just their comfort. And they must persevere through the inevitable missteps and false starts, cheering each other on until they find a solution.

Other cooperative challenges you could try:

- Group Storytelling: Players take turns adding one sentence at a time to a make-believe story, building on each other's ideas and steering the plot toward a satisfying conclusion.
- Blindfolded Obstacle Course: Set up a simple obstacle course in your living room or backyard. One child puts on a blindfold and tries to navigate the course with verbal guidance from their teammates.
- Balloon Keep-Up: The group tries to keep a balloon aloft for as long as possible, calling out each other's names to pass the balloon and strategizing to cover the whole space.
- Scavenger Hunt: Teams work together to find and photograph a list of objects or landmarks around the neighborhood, park, or house. Include riddles or clues that require group input to solve to encourage creative teamwork.

As a parent facilitator, your role is to introduce the activity, clarify any rules or safety guidelines, and then step back and let the kids lead. Avoid jumping in with solutions or critiques, even if you see a more efficient path forward. Learning happens through trial and error, the giving and taking of ideas, and the "aha" moments when a new approach clicks.

Instead, focus on reflecting on the group process as you observe it:

"I noticed how you all listened carefully to Jaden's idea and then built on it with your suggestions."

"It looked like you were getting frustrated for a minute there, but you took some deep breaths and kept trying different strategies until you found one that worked!"

"I saw a lot of high-fives and smiles when you finally reached your goal. How did it feel to overcome that challenge as a team?"

These specific, descriptive comments help kids tune into the concrete behaviors that lead to successful collaboration. By focusing on the process, not just the outcome, you emphasize that teamwork is an ongoing practice, not a fixed ability.

If conflicts or hurt feelings do arise during the game, resist the urge to swoop in and referee. Instead, ask open-ended questions that prompt kids to problem-solve together:

"What do you think happened there? How could we rewind and try that again in a way that feels good for everyone?"

"I hear two different wants - Maria wants to be the leader, and Jake wants a turn, too. What's a compromise that could work for both of you?"

By modeling curiosity and empowering kids to find their solutions, you foster the resilience and resourcefulness they need to navigate social challenges in the real world. You send the message that mistakes and disagreements are natural parts of working together, not catastrophes to be avoided at all costs.

Of course, cooperative play doesn't have to be all serious skill-building. Feel free to get silly and creative with your game designs! Challenge kids to build the tallest possible tower out of household objects, or put on a family talent show with each person contributing their unique flair. The more laughter and joy you bring to the process, the more kids will associate collaboration with positive connections.

As you make cooperative games a regular part of your family's play routine, you may start to notice subtle shifts in the way your kids approach social situations. They may pause to consider others' perspectives before barreling ahead with their agendas. They may suggest compromises or ask for help more readily when stuck on a homework problem. And they may bounce back more quickly from conflicts, knowing that repair and reconnection are always possible.

In a world that often pits us against each other in a race for individual success, the social skills learned through cooperative play are more vital than ever. By nurturing our kids' capacity for empathy, communication, and creative collaboration, we equip them to build a future of mutual understanding and collective flourishing. And that's the ultimate team victory.

EXERCISE 1: HELPING HANDS

Objective:

This activity teaches children how to offer and accept help graciously while practicing perspective-taking and empathy.

Materials:

- Scenario cards (see examples below)
- Open space for role-playing

Instructions:

1. Introduce the concept of helping hands by discussing what it means to offer and accept help. Brainstorm

examples of when someone might need help and how it feels to receive help.

2. Present a series of scenario cards that depict different situations where one person needs help and another person offers to assist them. For example:

- A child is struggling to carry a heavy backpack.
- A friend is having trouble understanding a math problem.
- A sibling is feeling upset after losing a game.
- A parent is running late and needs help getting ready.

3. Divide into pairs and assign each pair a scenario card. Give them a few minutes to discuss how they want to act out the scene, focusing on what the helper will say and do.

4. Have each pair take turns role-playing their scenario in front of the group. Encourage the "helper" to use kind words and body language, such as offering a smile, making eye contact, and using a gentle tone of voice.

5. After each role-play, discuss as a group what the helper did well and how the person being helped might have felt. Brainstorm alternative ways of offering help and responding to help.

6. Switch roles and have each pair role-play the scenario again, with the other person being the helper. Notice any differences in how help is offered or received.

7. Debrief as a group about what it was like to give and receive help. What makes it easier or harder to ask for help? How can we show appreciation when someone helps us?

Tips:
- Adapt the scenarios to your child's age and experiences. For younger children, focus on concrete, familiar situations. For older children, include more complex social dynamics.
- Model offering and accepting help in your interactions with your child and others. Point out examples of helping hands in books, movies, or real life.
- Encourage your child to look for opportunities to offer help in their daily life, such as holding the door for someone, picking up a dropped item, or offering to share a snack.
- Discuss the difference between helping and rescuing. Emphasize that true helping empowers the other person and respects their autonomy rather than doing everything for them.

EXERCISE 2: HUMAN KNOT

Objective:

This classic team-building activity promotes cooperation, problem-solving, and non-verbal communication as participants work together to untangle themselves from a human knot.

Materials:

- Open space large enough for your group to stand in a circle
- Optional: Blindfolds for an added challenge

Instructions:

1. Have all participants stand in a tight circle, facing inward. Encourage them to take a moment to make eye contact and smile at each other.

2. Ask each person to reach out their right hand and grab the hand of someone across the circle as if they are shaking hands. Make sure each person is holding the hand of a different person.

3. Next, have each person reach out their left hand and grab the hand of a different person across the circle. Double-check that everyone is holding the hands of two different people and that no one is holding the hands of someone directly beside them.

4. Explain that the goal of the game is to untangle the human knot and re-form the circle without anyone letting go of the hands they are holding. The group must work together to figure out how to twist, turn, and step over or under each other's arms to untangle the knot.

5. Encourage participants to go slowly and carefully, communicating with each other through words and body language. Remind them to be gentle and respectful of each other's bodies and personal space.

6. If the group gets stuck, offer suggestions or hints, such as having one person be a leader and guide the others through the untangling process. If the knot seems impossible to untangle, allow participants to let go and start over.

7. Once the group has successfully untangled the knot and re-formed the circle, celebrate their achievement and reflect on the experience. What strategies did they use to communicate and cooperate? What was challenging or frustrating about the process?

Tips:

- For an added challenge, try the activity in silence, using only non-verbal communication to guide the untangling process. Or have participants wear blindfolds and rely on verbal instructions from a designated leader.
- Discuss the importance of trust, patience, and persistence in teamwork. How can participants apply these skills in other areas of their lives, such as group projects or family challenges?
- If you have a large group, divide it into smaller circles of 8-10 people each. You can have the small groups compete to see who can untangle their knot the fastest or work together as a mega-team to solve a giant knot.

- Adapt the activity for children with mobility challenges by having them sit in a circle and use string or ribbon to create the knot rather than their arms and hands.

EXERCISE 3: MINEFIELD

Objective:

This activity builds trust, communication, and active listening skills as partners navigate a challenging obstacle course together.

Materials:

- Large open spaces, such as a room, yard, or park
- Blindfolds or sleep masks for each pair
- Various obstacles, such as cones, balls, stuffed animals, hula hoops, etc.

Instructions:

1. Set up a "minefield" obstacle course in your open space using the various objects you have gathered. Spread the obstacles out in a random pattern, with enough space between them for a person to walk through.

2. Divide participants into pairs and give each pair a blindfold or sleep mask. Explain that one partner will be wearing the blindfold and navigating the minefield while the other partner will be giving verbal instructions to guide them through safely.

3. Have each pair decide who will be the navigator and who will be the traveler first. The traveler should put on the blindfold and stand at the edge of the minefield while the navigator stands outside the course where they can see the whole area.

4. Explain that the goal is for the traveler to make it through the minefield without touching any of the obstacles, relying solely on the verbal instructions of their navigator. The navigator cannot enter the minefield or touch the traveler; they can only use their words to guide and direct.

5. Give the pairs a few minutes to discuss their communication strategy, such as what specific words or directions they will use. Encourage them to agree on a "stop" signal in case the traveler feels unsafe or needs to pause.

6. Have each pair take turns navigating the minefield, with the navigator offering clear, concise instructions and the traveler listening carefully and following the directions. Encourage the navigator to use descriptive language and spatial cues, such as "take two steps forward" or "turn 90 degrees to your left."

7. If the traveler touches an obstacle, they must go back to the start and try again. The navigator can adjust their instructions based on what they observed the first time.

8. After each pair has had a turn navigating the minefield, debrief as a group about the experience. What was it like to trust and rely on someone else's guidance? What made the communication effective or challenging?

Tips:

- Adapt the difficulty of the minefield based on the age and abilities of your group. For younger children, use fewer and larger obstacles. For older children or adults, create a more complex course with multiple pathways.
- Discuss the importance of giving and receiving feedback constructively. How can the navigator offer guidance and support without being bossy or critical? How can the traveler ask for clarification or express their needs and limits?
- Extend the activity by having pairs navigate real-world "minefields," such as a crowded hallway or a busy street crossing. Discuss how they can apply their communication and trust skills in these situations.
- Emphasize the value of active listening and paying attention to non-verbal cues, such as tone of voice and body language. How can participants use all their senses to understand and respond to their partner's needs?

CHAPTER 15: SUPPORTING EMOTIONAL AWARENESS AND VALIDATION THROUGH PLAY

MODELING EMOTIONAL LITERACY DURING PLAY INTERACTIONS

Imagine a world where feelings had no names. Where the tightness in your chest when you're anxious, the heat rising in your cheeks when you're embarrassed, or the electric joy buzzing through your body when you're excited had no labels to contain them. For young children, this nameless swirl of sensations and reactions is their daily reality. They experience a rollercoaster of emotions but lack the vocabulary to articulate them, leaving them feeling overwhelmed and alone.

One of the greatest gifts you can offer your child as a parent is the language of emotional literacy. By consistently labeling and validating the full spectrum of feelings that arise during play, you help your child develop a robust repertoire for understanding and expressing their inner world. You teach them that all emotions are normal, manageable, and worthy of being seen and heard.

The beauty of the play is that it naturally evokes a kaleidoscope of feelings that might not surface in everyday conversations. A child who presents as calm and compliant in the classroom may suddenly erupt in frustration when their block tower keeps tumbling down. A child who hides their hurts behind a joking facade may act out a poignant story of a lonely kitten searching for a friend. By attuning to these unspoken emotions and reflecting them with empathy, you create a safe space for your child to explore the peaks and valleys of their inner landscape.

Here are some examples of how you might model emotional validation during play:

- "Wow, that dinosaur looks really mad! His face is all scrunched up, and his fists are clenched tight. It must be so frustrating to keep getting knocked down by the T-Rex."
- "I noticed your voice got very soft, and your shoulders slumped down when the doll said she didn't want to play anymore. That must have felt so sad and lonely."
- "Your eyes are shining, and you're bouncing up and down with a huge smile! Building that rocket ship all by yourself must make you feel so proud and excited!"
- "That tiger cub is crying and hiding in the cave. He seems really scared to go out and face that loud noise. I wonder what would help him feel safe and brave again?"

Notice how these reflective statements focus on naming the specific emotions and body language cues you observe without judgment or minimizing. Rather than rushing to reassure or problem-solve, you acknowledge and accept your child's feeling state, inviting them to elaborate if they wish. You follow their lead and resist projecting your assumptions onto the play narrative.

This language of emotional attunement may feel stilted or awkward at first, especially if you grew up in a family where feelings were rarely discussed. But with practice, you'll find that it becomes a natural, intuitive way of connecting with your child on a heart level. You'll discover the magic of simply being present and bearing witness to their emotional truth, trusting in their innate resilience and capacity for self-regulation.

Of course, some emotions may feel too big or scary for your child to process alone. When intense feelings like rage, despair, or terror threaten to overwhelm your child, they need more than just validation - they need your calm, grounded presence to help them weather the storm. In these moments, it's okay to offer a soothing touch, co-regulating breaths, or gentle redirection to a more structured activity. But even then, keep affirming the emotion itself as valid and understandable given the circumstances.

As you model emotional literacy and acceptance during play, you may be amazed at how readily your child begins to adopt this language themselves. They may start narrating their doll's frustration at getting dressed or labeling their disappointment when a game doesn't go their way. They may become more curious about the nuances of their own and others' feeling states, asking questions like "How do you know when you're feeling jealous?" or "What helps you calm down when you're really mad?"

This budding emotional self-awareness is a crucial building block for mental health and relationship success. By learning to recognize, name, and respond to their feelings, children develop a secure sense of self and the tools to navigate life's inevitable ups and downs. And by internalizing a template for empathetic listening, they lay the groundwork for deep, authentic connections with others.

So keep sprinkling those play moments with emotional color commentary and curiosity. Keep showing up for your child's inner world with an open, accepting heart. With every "You seem so excited!" or "That part made you feel really angry, huh?", you are planting seeds of self-love and resilience that will bear fruit for a lifetime.

PLAYFUL ACTIVITIES FOR EXPLORING EMOTIONS AND BUILDING COPING SKILLS

Emotional literacy is not just about naming feelings but also learning how to express and regulate them in healthy ways. For children who are still developing impulse control and communication skills, this can be a tall order. They may lash out when upset, bottle up their anger until it explodes, or shut down and withdraw when overwhelmed. The play offers a powerful medium to practice identifying emotions, understanding their triggers, and experimenting with coping strategies in a safe, fun context.

Here are some playful activities that can help expand your child's emotional repertoire:

1. *Feelings Charades:* Write different emotions on slips of paper and take turns acting them out silently while the other person guesses. For an added challenge, include subtler feeling states like "nervous," "disappointed," or "confused." This game builds emotional vocabulary and non-verbal communication skills.

2. *Emoji Check-Ins:* Print out a sheet of emoji faces representing various emotions. At regular intervals during play (or throughout the day), invite your child to point to the emoji that best matches their current mood. Use this as a springboard to discuss what's contributing to their feeling state and brainstorm coping strategies if needed.

3. ***Calming Toolkit:*** Work with your child to decorate a shoebox or bag and fill it with soothing objects and activities that engage their five senses. Some ideas: lavender playdough, a glitter jar, squishy stress balls, coloring pages, bubbles, and a soft stuffed animal. Please encourage them to choose an item from their toolkit when they need help calming down.

4. ***Mood Music:*** Create a playlist together with songs that evoke different emotions - from upbeat dance tunes to soulful ballads. Take turns playing "DJ" and see if you can guess each other's mood based on their song choice. Discuss how music can shift or intensify feeling states and which songs help you feel better when you're down.

5. ***Feelings Forecast:*** Challenge your child to create a "weather report" for their emotions, using metaphors like "sunny skies," "partly cloudy," or "thunderstorms." Encourage them to get creative with their descriptions and to identify the "fronts" moving in or out of their emotional atmosphere. This activity promotes self-reflection and symbolic thinking.

6. ***Emotion Potions:*** Gather clear glass jars, food coloring, glitter, and small trinkets. Have your child choose colors and objects to represent different emotions, then mix them with water in the jars. As they stir, invite them to imagine the feelings swirling and transforming. Use this as a visual aid to discuss how emotions can blend, change, or settle over time.

7. ***Feelings Jenga:*** Using a Jenga set or tumbling block tower, take turns pulling out blocks and answering the questions written on them. Include prompts like "What makes you feel scared? " "How do you show love? " or "When was a time you felt really proud of yourself?" This game sparks emotional reflection while building frustration tolerance.

8. ***Worry Box:*** Decorate a small box together and invite your child to write or draw their worries on slips of paper to put inside. Set a regular time (e.g., before bed) to pull out one worry at a time and discuss solutions or coping strategies. This externalizes concerns and builds problem-solving skills.

Remember, the goal of these activities is not to eliminate or fix negative emotions but to normalize them as part of the human experience. Please encourage your child to approach their feelings with curiosity and compassion rather than judgment or avoidance. Model healthy coping strategies like deep breathing, positive self-talk, or seeking support when you're struggling.

If your child resists these playful interventions at first, don't force it. Some kids may feel self-conscious about acting out emotions or prefer to process feelings privately. Focus on creating an overall environment of emotional safety and acceptance, trusting that your child will open up when they're ready.

The most powerful emotional lessons often happen in the unplanned, organic moments of play and connection. When you join your child in a tickle fight and validate their joy or snuggle them through tears of disappointment, you are teaching them that their feelings matter. You are showing them that even the messiest emotions can be held with tenderness and care.

As your child grows more fluent in the language of emotion, you may find them naturally incorporating their new skills into everyday interactions. They may take a deep breath before tackling a frustrating homework assignment or express empathy for a friend who is struggling. They may use "I feel" statements to assert their needs rather than lashing out or shutting down.

These small victories are the true measure of emotional intelligence - not just knowing the right words but living them out in real-world relationships. And it all starts with the playful, loving exchanges you share in the haven of your connection. So keep making space for the full rainbow of feelings in your child's play world, and watch as they blossom into a resilient, empathetic force for good.

EXERCISE 1: EMO-LIBS

Objective:

This activity builds emotional vocabulary and self-expression by having participants fill in blank spaces in a story or song with different feeling words and acting them out.

Materials:

- Emo-Libs templates (see examples below)
- Pencils or pens
- Optional: Props or costumes for acting out the stories

Instructions:

1. Introduce the concept of Emo-Libs by showing an example of a familiar story or song with the feeling words blanked out. Explain that participants will be creating their versions by filling in the blanks with different emotions.

2. Provide a selection of Emo-Libs templates, such as:

  - "Old MacDonald had a ____ (feeling) farm."

  - "The Three ____ (feeling) Bears"

  - "If You're ____ (feeling) and You Know It"

  - "I Feel ____ (feeling) When You're Gone"

3. Have participants choose a template and fill in the blank spaces with feeling words of their choice. Encourage them to use a variety of emotions, both comfortable and uncomfortable.

4. Invite participants to share their completed Emo-Libs with the group by reading them aloud with dramatic flair. Encourage them to use facial expressions, body language, and tone of voice to convey their chosen emotions.

5. After each share, discuss how the inserted feelings changed the meaning or tone of the story/song. What would it be like to experience that particular mix of emotions? How might the characters respond differently

based on their feelings?

6. Choose one or two Emo-Libs to act out as a group, assigning roles and using props or costumes as desired. Ham it up and exaggerate the emotional expressions for a playful effect.

7. Debrief the activity by reflecting on how it felt to name and express different emotions in a creative context. What did participants notice about the range and nuance of feelings available? How can they apply this emotional awareness in real life?

Example Emo-Libs template:

Once upon a time, there was a ____ (feeling) princess who lived in a ____ (feeling) castle. One day, a ____ (feeling) dragon came to the castle and said, "I'm feeling ____ (feeling), and I need your help!" The princess felt ____ (feeling), but she agreed to help the dragon. Together, they went on a ____ (feeling) journey and learned that it's okay to feel ____ (feeling) sometimes. In the end, they both felt ____ (feeling) and lived happily ever after.

Tips:

- Provide a feelings word bank for younger children or those who need extra support with emotional vocabulary. Include a mix of basic and complex feelings, such as happy, sad, angry, excited, nervous, frustrated, proud, disappointed, etc.
- Encourage participants to think beyond just "positive" or "negative" emotions and explore the full spectrum of feelings. Validate all emotional experiences as normal and okay.
- Discuss how different characters in the same story might have different emotional reactions based on their perspectives and experiences. Promote empathy and perspective-taking.
- Create your own Emo-Libs templates based on your child's favorite books, movies, or songs. You can also have them write their own stories with blank spaces for feelings.

EXERCISE 2: FEELINGS FEAST

Objective:

This activity promotes emotional awareness and regulation by having participants imagine and describe feeling foods and then practice "digesting" them through mindful breathing.

Materials:

- Paper plates or placemats
- Markers or crayons
- Optional: Real or toy food items

Instructions:

1. Introduce the concept of a Feelings Feast by explaining that just like we need to eat a variety of foods to

nourish our bodies, we need to experience and express a variety of emotions to nourish our minds and hearts.

2. Give each participant a paper plate or placemat and some markers/crayons. Invite them to imagine they are at a buffet filled with feeling foods, where each dish represents a different emotion.

3. Have participants draw or list the feeling foods they would like to "eat" at this imaginary feast. Encourage them to include a mix of comfortable and uncomfortable emotions, such as:

- Happy hamburgers
- Sad spaghetti
- Angry apples
- Excited eggs
- Nervous noodles
- Proud pizza
- Disappointed dumplings

4. Invite participants to share their feeling-food plates with the group, describing what each dish represents and why they chose it. Validate all emotional experiences as normal and okay.

5. Discuss how different feeling foods might "taste" or "feel" in our bodies. Where do we feel them? What sensations or thoughts come up? How long do they "stay with us"?

6. Have participants choose one feeling food to "eat" and imagine chewing it slowly, noticing all the flavors and textures. Guide them to take deep breaths as they "digest" the feeling, sending it to different parts of their body.

7. Practice "digesting" a few different feeling foods through mindful breathing, emphasizing that all emotions are meant to be felt and processed, not avoided or judged.

8. Debrief the activity by discussing how we can "nourish" ourselves with a balanced diet of emotions, neither stuffing ourselves with too much of one feeling nor starving ourselves of important emotional experiences.

Tips:

- Use real or toy food items to make the activity more concrete and engaging for younger children. Have them arrange the foods on their plate and practice naming the associated feelings.
- Discuss how some feeling foods might be an "acquired taste" that we need to try multiple times before we develop a liking for them. Emphasize the value of staying open and curious about all emotional experiences.
- Explore the idea of "comfort foods" that we turn to when we're feeling down and how we can find healthy ways to soothe and nourish ourselves emotionally.
- Extend the activity by having participants create a "feelings menu" with different emotional dishes for different occasions, such as a "bravery burrito" for facing fear or a "calm cupcake" for winding down before bed.

EXERCISE 3: EMOJI MASKS

Objective:

This activity builds emotional expression and empathy by having participants create and wear masks depicting different feeling faces and then practice responding to each other's emotional states.

Materials:

- Paper plates or pre-cut mask templates
- Markers, crayons, or other decorating materials
- Scissors
- String or elastic for attaching masks
- Optional: Emotion prompt cards

Instructions:

1. Introduce the concept of emoji masks by showing examples of different emotional expressions, either in digital emoji form or on real human faces. Discuss how our facial expressions communicate our feelings to others.

2. Give each participant a paper plate or mask template and decorating materials. Invite them to create 3-4 different masks, each depicting a different emotion, such as happy, sad, angry, surprised, scared, confused, etc.

3. Have participants cut out eye holes and attach string or elastic to their masks so they can wear them.

4. Introduce the idea of "emotional charades" by having participants take turns wearing one of their masks and acting out a scene or situation that might evoke that feeling. The rest of the group tries to guess the emotion based on facial expressions and body language.

5. Discuss how we can "read" other people's emotional states based on their nonverbal cues and how this skill helps us respond with empathy and care. Practice making different feeling faces and noting the subtle differences between similar emotions.

6. Have participants break into pairs and take turns wearing their masks while the other person practices responding with empathy and validation. Encourage them to use reflective listening statements, such as "It looks like you're feeling really sad right now" or "I can see how angry that situation made you."

7. Use emotional prompt cards to guide the role-plays, such as "Your best friend canceled your playdate" or "You got a perfect score on your math test." Discuss how different people might have different emotional reactions to the same situation.

8. Debrief the activity by reflecting on how it felt to express and respond to different emotions through the masks. What did participants notice about the power of nonverbal communication? How can they apply this awareness in their daily interactions?

Tips:

- Provide a feelings word bank or chart to help participants name and differentiate between different emotions. Encourage them to be specific and nuanced in their descriptions.

- Discuss the difference between "showing" an emotion and "becoming" it. Emphasize that we can express and empathize with feelings without being controlled by them.
- Have participants create masks for complex or mixed emotions, such as "nervoucited" (nervous + excited) or "hangry" (hungry + angry). Discuss how we often feel multiple emotions at once and how to navigate these experiences.
- Extend the activity by having participants create masks for different "parts" of themselves, such as their "wise self," "fearful self," or "playful self." Use these masks to role-play internal dialogues and self-compassion.

EXERCISE 4: EMPATHY CHARADES

Objective:

This activity promotes empathy and perspective-taking by having participants act out challenging situations and respond with validating statements.

Materials:

- Scenario cards (see examples below)
- Timer or phone
- Optional: Props or costumes for acting

Instructions:

1. Introduce the concept of empathy as the ability to understand and share the feelings of another person. Discuss why empathy is important for building caring relationships and communities.

2. Explain the rules of Empathy Charades:

- One person (the actor) will draw a scenario card and act out the situation using body language and facial expressions but no words.
- The rest of the group (the empathizers) will try to guess what the actor is feeling and offer validating responses.
- The actor can give a thumbs up or down to indicate if the empathizers are on the right track.
- Once the feeling is correctly guessed, the empathizers take turns offering verbal validations and support.

3. Provide a set of scenario cards that depict common challenging situations for children, such as:

- You're left out of a game at recess.
- Your favorite toy breaks.
- You have to give a presentation in front of the class.
- Your parents are arguing.
- You get a bad grade on a test.
- A friend doesn't invite you to their birthday party.

4. Have participants take turns being the actors and the empathizers. Set a timer for 1-2 minutes per round to keep the activity moving.

5. Encourage the empathizers to use validating statements that name the feeling and show understanding, such as:

- "That must have been really embarrassing."
- "It's so frustrating when something doesn't go the way you wanted."
- "I can see how much that hurt your feelings."
- "It's okay to feel scared; I'm here for you."

6. Discuss how it feels to receive empathy and validation when you're going through a tough time. What kind of responses are most helpful or comforting?

7. Debrief the activity by reflecting on how participants can apply empathy skills in their daily lives. Brainstorm ways to show compassion and care for others who are struggling.

Tips:

- Model empathetic responses during the game to help participants learn the language of validation. Avoid jumping to problem-solving or silver linings; focus on acknowledging the feeling first.
- Discuss the difference between empathy and sympathy. Empathy is feeling "with" someone, while sympathy is feeling "for" them. Empathy involves a deeper level of understanding and connection.
- Have participants brainstorm their scenario cards based on real-life challenges they've faced. Discuss how empathy can help build resilience and coping skills.
- Extend the activity by having participants write empathy notes or create care packages for someone who is going through a difficult time. Encourage them to use their empathy skills to offer comfort and support.

Remember, emotional intelligence is a key foundation for mental health and thriving relationships. By creating playful opportunities for children to build emotional awareness, expression, and empathy, you equip them with the tools they need to navigate life's ups and downs with resilience and compassion. So have fun, get creative, and celebrate the power of emotions!

CHAPTER 16: BUILDING DISTRESS TOLERANCE THROUGH STRATEGIC PLAY CHOICES

ENCOURAGING PERSEVERANCE AND RESILIENCE THROUGH CHALLENGING PLAY

In today's instant gratification culture, it's easy for kids to get frustrated and give up when a task doesn't yield immediate results. From fast-loading videos to same-day delivery, children are accustomed to having their needs met with a swipe or a click. But as any adult knows, real life is full of challenges that require patience, persistence, and creative problem-solving. Luckily, playtime offers an ideal training ground for building these vital skills of resilience.

By intentionally choosing toys and games that present an optimal level of difficulty, parents can help children develop a growth mindset—the belief that abilities can be strengthened through effort and learning. Rather than shielding kids from struggle, strategic challenges teach them to embrace the process of trial and error, see setbacks as opportunities for growth, and persevere in the face of frustration.

Take puzzles, for instance. Piecing together a 100-piece jigsaw may seem like an exercise in futility to a child who is used to the instant feedback of digital games. They may quickly lose interest or declare it "too hard" at the first sign of difficulty. But with encouragement and subtle guidance, that same child can learn to break the daunting task into smaller chunks, try different strategies like sorting by color or finding the edge pieces, and celebrate each incremental victory.

As they work through the inevitable stuck points and "aha" moments, they are not just exercising their spatial reasoning and fine motor control - they are building mental muscles of focus, flexible thinking, and distress tolerance. They are learning that success often requires sustained effort, that mistakes are part of the process, and that their grit and ingenuity can carry them through tough challenges.

Other toys and games that can promote perseverance and problem-solving:

- Brain teasers and logic puzzles
- Rubik's cubes and other 3D manipulatives
- Construction sets like LEGO or K'NEX
- Strategy board games like chess or Risk
- Open-ended building materials like blocks or magna tiles
- Mechanical models and science kits
- Elaborately themed dollhouses or action figure sets

The key is to choose activities that are just challenging enough to keep your child engaged without tipping into frustration overload. Vygotsky's concept of the "zone of proximal development" offers a useful framework here - aim for tasks that your child can't quite master independently but can succeed at with some scaffolding and support.

As a play partner, your role is to provide encouragement and gentle guidance while resisting the urge to swoop in and solve problems for your child. This may mean biting your tongue when you see an easier solution, offering hints rather than direct answers, or modeling coping strategies like taking a deep breath or trying a new angle.

Some prompts you might try when your child gets stuck:

- "You've tried so many different ideas! What else could you try?"
- "It's okay to feel frustrated. Let's take a break and come back with fresh eyes."
- "Mistakes help us learn. What can we change for next time?"
- "This is a tough one! How could we break it down into smaller steps?"
- "I see you working so hard. You're really sticking with it!"

Notice how these statements validate your child's effort and emotions while also emphasizing their agency in finding solutions. By framing challenges as opportunities for learning and growth, you help your child develop an internal locus of control - the belief that they have the power to influence outcomes through their actions.

Of course, it's important to balance challenging play with plenty of free, unstructured exploration as well. Children need ample time to let their minds wander, to invent their games and stories, and to process the day's stresses and stimulations. Pretend play, in particular, offers a rich landscape for developing emotional resilience and flexibility.

In the next section, we'll explore how imaginative scenarios can help children practice acceptance and letting go in the face of change and disappointment. Through the safe distance of make-believe, kids can grapple with life's bittersweet realities and emerge with greater perspective and adaptability.

INTRODUCING ACCEPTANCE AND LETTING GO THROUGH IMAGINATIVE PLAY

Change is a constant in children's lives, from the daily rhythms of separating from caregivers to the seismic shifts of moving homes or welcoming new siblings. Kids may also face acute losses like the death of a pet, the departure of a friend, or the ending of a beloved activity. Even positive transitions like graduating from preschool or mastering a new skill require letting go of familiar routines and identities.

For children who thrive on predictability and control, these changes can feel overwhelming and unfair. They may resist or deny painful realities, clinging to the way things were with all their might. While this desire for stability is natural and adaptive, learning to accept and adapt to life's inevitable fluctuations is a key task of healthy development.

Pretend play offers a powerful tool for exploring themes of change, loss, and impermanence in a safe, symbolic space. By acting out characters and stories that grapple with transitions and goodbyes, children can metabolize their own mixed emotions and experiment with coping strategies at a distance. They can project their fears and wishes onto the play narrative, testing out different endings and meanings.

Here are some ways you can subtly introduce these themes into your child's imaginative play:

- Create a story about a character saying goodbye to a beloved toy or security object before a big move. What helps them feel brave and remember the good times?

- Set up a play scene in which a magical land undergoes a seasonal change, like winter melting into spring. How do the creatures adapt to the new environment? What do they miss and look forward to?
- Enact a scenario where a child's favorite superhero is retiring and passing the torch to a new hero. How does the old hero feel about this transition? What wisdom do they impart to their successor?
- Imagine a world where people trade in their old dreams for new ones at a special shop. What kinds of dreams do they let go of and why? What hopes and fears do they have about embracing a new vision?

As you play out these symbolic narratives, use validation and mindfulness language to model acknowledging difficult feelings without judgment:

- "It's so hard to say goodbye to Bear. You two have been through so much together. It's okay to feel sad and scared."
- "The flowers and trees look confused by the new weather. They miss the warm sun, but they're also curious about what spring will bring."
- "I can see Hero feeling proud of all his adventures but also a little lost without his cape. Retiring is bittersweet like that."
- "Choosing a new dream takes a lot of courage. It's normal to worry if you're making the right choice. What helps Dream Giver trust her heart?"

Notice how these reflections make space for the full range of emotions that come with change - the grief and anxiety alongside the excitement and hope. By giving voice to these conflicting feelings through the characters' experiences, you help your child build a vocabulary for their inner world. You show them that all their reactions are valid and speakable, even the messy, confusing ones.

At the same time, you can gently model perspectives and coping strategies that promote resilience and acceptance:

- "Bear will always be in your heart, even when you can't hug him. What special memories will you carry with you?"
- "The creatures are finding new ways to have fun in the snow - sledding, building forts, sipping hot cocoa. What other winter joys could they discover?"
- "Hero is excited to share his wisdom with the next generation. Teaching feels like a new kind of superpower!"
- "Dream Giver is grateful for all her old dreams taught her. She knows each one prepared her for this new adventure."

By embodying these growth-oriented attitudes through play, you help your child internalize a sense of continuity and meaning amidst life's upheavals. They learn that change, while difficult, can also bring new opportunities and insights. They discover their capacity to carry forward what matters most while also embracing the unknown.

This emotional flexibility is a key ingredient of resilience - the ability to adapt and thrive in the face of adversity. When children know in their bones that loss and transition are survivable, even generative, they can meet life's challenges with greater stability and resourcefulness. They can grieve what's ended while also leaning into what's beginning.

Of course, no amount of pretend play can shield kids from the pain of real-world goodbyes and disappointments. There will still be times when your child rails against an unwanted change or dissolves into tears at a bittersweet ending. In these moments, your loving presence and empathetic attunement are the ultimate anchors.

By sitting with your child in the discomfort of hard feelings, you teach them that their grief is not shameful or too much for you to handle. By reminiscing about what's been lost and wondering about what's to come, you model a spirit of open acceptance and curiosity. And by trusting your child's innate resilience and creativity, you empower them to find their path forward, even in the darkest of times.

So keep weaving those themes of change and growth into your child's play, and watch as they gradually learn to surf life's unpredictable waves with greater confidence and grace. With each symbolic goodbye and a new beginning, they are internalizing a template for navigating loss and transition that will serve them long into adulthood. And with your unconditional love and support, they are building an unshakeable foundation of inner security that can weather any storm.

EXERCISE 1: CALM DOWN CUBE

Objective:

This activity teaches children a variety of coping strategies to use when they are feeling overwhelmed or distressed, using a playful, tactile tool.

Materials:

- Blank cube template (can be found online or made from scratch)
- Markers, crayons, or stickers for decorating
- Scissors
- Tape or glue

Instructions:

1. Introduce the concept of distress tolerance as the ability to cope with difficult emotions or situations without making things worse. Discuss why it's important to have a variety of strategies to use when we're feeling upset.

2. Show an example of a Calm Down Cube, with each side labeled with a different coping skill, such as:

- Take 5 deep breaths
- Count backwards from 10
- Do a silly dance
- Say a positive affirmation
- Squeeze a stress ball
- Ask for a hug

3. Provide each participant with a blank cube template and decorating materials. Invite them to fill in each side of the cube with a different coping strategy that they find helpful or want to try.

4. Encourage participants to get creative with their designs, using colors, patterns, or pictures that make them feel calm or happy. They can also add their unique strategies or variations on the examples provided.

5. Have participants cut out and assemble their cubes using tape or glue. Demonstrate how to roll the cube and practice the strategy that lands on top.

6. Discuss when and how participants can use their Calm Down Cubes, such as during a frustrating homework assignment, after a fight with a friend, or when they're feeling anxious about a new situation.

7. Have participants take turns rolling their cubes and demonstrating the strategies for the group. Provide feedback and encouragement as they practice each skill.

8. Debrief the activity by reflecting on how it feels to have a tangible tool for coping with distress. What strategies do participants think will be most helpful for them? How can they remember to use their cubes in the moment of upset?

Tips:

- Provide a list of suggested coping strategies for participants who may have trouble generating their ideas. Include a mix of sensory, cognitive, and physical activities.
- Discuss how different strategies may work better for different types of distress. For example, deep breathing may be helpful for anxiety, while distraction may be better for anger.
- Encourage participants to keep their Calm Down Cubes in a visible, accessible place, such as on their desk or bedside table. They can also make mini versions to carry in their pocket or backpack.
- Have participants practice using their cubes during calm times so they are more likely to remember and use them during times of distress. Reinforce their efforts with praise and encouragement.

EXERCISE 2: COPING SKILLS TOOLKIT

Objective:

This activity helps children create a personalized collection of sensory objects and activity cards to use when they are feeling dysregulated or overwhelmed.

Materials:

- Small box, bag, or container for each participant
- Various sensory fidgets and stress-relief objects, such as:
- Stress balls or squishy toys
- Fidget spinners or cubes
- Rubber bands or stretchy strings
- Soft fabrics or stuffed animals
- Essential oils or scented playdough
- Chewing gum or crunchy snacks
- Index cards or cardstock
- Writing and drawing utensils

Instructions:

1. Introduce the concept of a Coping Skills Toolkit as a collection of objects and activities that can help us calm down and cope with difficult emotions. Discuss how different people may find different things helpful based on their unique sensory preferences and interests.

2. Provide a variety of sensory objects and fidgets for participants to explore. Encourage them to notice how each item feels, looks, sounds, smells, or tastes and what kind of emotional response it evokes.

3. Invite participants to choose 3-5 objects that they find most soothing or engaging to include in their Coping Skills Toolkit. Provide a small box, bag, or container for them to store their items.

4. Have participants create a set of activity cards to include in their toolkit, with each card depicting a different coping strategy or pleasant distraction, such as:

- Listen to calming music
- Color or draw a picture
- Write in a journal
- Do a puzzle or brain teaser
- Play with a favorite toy
- Talk to a trusted friend or adult

5. Encourage participants to decorate their activity cards and containers to make them visually appealing and personalized. They can also add their unique coping ideas or resources, such as photos of loved ones or inspiring quotes.

6. Have participants practice using their Coping Skills Toolkits in a variety of scenarios, such as when they are feeling anxious, angry, sad, or bored. Discuss how different tools or activities may be more or less helpful depending on the situation.

7. Brainstorm ways to make the Coping Skills Toolkit easily accessible and portable, such as keeping it in a special spot at home or school or creating a mini version to carry in a pocket or backpack.

8. Debrief the activity by reflecting on how it feels to have a personalized set of resources for coping with distress. What was the process of creating the toolkit like? How do participants plan to use and update their toolkits over time?

Tips:

- Provide a wide range of sensory options to accommodate different preferences and needs. Some participants may prefer visual stimuli, while others may respond better to tactile or auditory input.
- Encourage participants to think outside the box when generating coping ideas. Activities can range from physical exercise to creative expression to social connection.
- Have participants practice using their toolkits during calm times so they are more familiar and comfortable with the items and activities when they need them most.
- Create a group or class Coping Skills Toolkit that participants can contribute to and borrow from as needed. This can help build a sense of community and support around emotional regulation.

EXERCISE 3: EMOTIONAL ENDURANCE CHALLENGE

Objective:

This activity helps children build distress tolerance by practicing persisting through a challenging or frustrating task in order to earn a reward.

Materials:

- Challenging puzzle, game, or activity that can be completed in 10-20 minutes
- Timer
- Small rewards or prizes
- Optional: Distress tolerance cards with coping strategies

Instructions:

1. Introduce the concept of emotional endurance as the ability to tolerate difficult feelings and sensations in order to reach a goal or complete a task. Discuss why this skill is important for success and well-being.

2. Present participants with a challenging puzzle, game, or activity that is slightly above their current skill level. Explain that the goal is to work on the task for a set amount of time (e.g., 15 minutes) without giving up, even if they feel frustrated or discouraged.

3. Set a timer for the designated work period and have participants begin the task. Encourage them to notice any difficult emotions or body sensations that arise, such as boredom, irritation, or restlessness.

4. If participants start to get dysregulated or want to quit, offer them a distress tolerance card with a coping strategy to try, such as:

- Take a deep breath and count to 10
- Do 10 jumping jacks or push-ups
- Say a positive self-statement, like "I can do this" or "This feeling will pass"
- Take a brief sensory break with a fidget or stress ball
- Visualize a peaceful or happy place
- Break the task into smaller steps and focus on one at a time

5. When the timer goes off, have participants stop working and celebrate their efforts, regardless of how much they completed. Emphasize the value of persistence and grit in the face of challenges.

6. Offer a small reward or prize for participants who were able to stick with the task for the full-time period. Discuss how the anticipation of a reward can help motivate us to push through difficult moments.

7. Have participants reflect on their experience with the Emotional Endurance Challenge. What emotions and sensations did they notice? What strategies helped them cope with the discomfort? How can they apply this skill in other areas of their life?

8. Repeat the activity with different tasks and longer periods to build participants' emotional endurance over time. Encourage them to track their progress and celebrate their growth.

Tips:

- Choose tasks that are challenging but not impossible to avoid feelings of helplessness or defeat. The goal is to build a sense of mastery and self-efficacy.
- Allow participants to take brief breaks or use coping strategies as needed, but encourage them to return to the task as soon as they feel able.
- Discuss the concept of "urge surfing," or riding out intense emotions or cravings without acting on them. Emphasize that difficult feelings are temporary and will eventually pass.
- Have participants create their Emotional Endurance Challenges based on their personal goals or areas of struggle. They can enlist a friend or family member to provide support and accountability.

EXERCISE 4: LETTING GO BUBBLES

Objective:

This activity teaches children to release stress and worries through the simple, playful act of blowing bubbles.

Materials:

- Bubble solution and wands (store-bought or homemade)
- Optional: Bubble-themed relaxation script or music

Instructions:

1. Introduce the concept of letting go as the ability to release thoughts, feelings, or situations that are no longer serving us. Discuss how holding onto stress or worries can weigh us down and keep us stuck.

2. Show participants how to use the bubble wands to blow bubbles, emphasizing the importance of taking a deep breath and exhaling slowly and steadily.

3. Invite participants to think of a worry, stress, or difficult situation that they would like to let go of. Encourage them to visualize this concern as a bubble, with all the associated thoughts and feelings contained inside.

4. Have participants take a deep breath in, imagining that they are filling their bubble with their stress or worry. As they exhale and blow through the wand, encourage them to imagine releasing the bubble and watching it float away.

5. Repeat the process with additional concerns or worries, emphasizing the sense of lightness and relief that comes with each release.

6. Encourage participants to notice the sensations of bubble-blowing, such as the cool air on their faces, the sticky solution on their fingers, and the shimmery colors of the bubbles. Discuss how focusing on these sensory details can help ground them in the present moment.

7. Have participants experiment with different types of bubbles, such as small, rapid-fire bubbles or giant, slow-moving bubbles. Discuss how the size and speed of the bubbles can reflect the intensity or duration of different worries or stresses.

8. End the activity with a few minutes of free bubble play, encouraging participants to enjoy the simple pleasure of creating and popping bubbles. You can play soft, relaxing music or read a bubble-themed relaxation script to

enhance the calming atmosphere.

9. Debrief the activity by reflecting on how it felt to release worries through the bubble-blowing. What did participants notice about their mind and body as they let go of each concern? How can they apply this letting go practice to other areas of their life?

Tips:

- Make your bubble solution by mixing 1 cup of water, 2 tablespoons of dish soap, and 1 tablespoon of glycerin or corn syrup. This creates stronger, longer-lasting bubbles.
- Have participants create their bubble wands using pipe cleaners, straws, or other materials. Encourage them to experiment with different shapes and sizes to see how they affect the bubbles.
- Do the activity outside on a breezy day to enhance the sense of release and freedom. Discuss how the wind can carry our worries away and disperse them into the larger world.
- Have participants write down their worries or stresses on slips of paper, then dissolve the papers in the bubble solution. As they blow bubbles, they can imagine their concerns literally dissolving and dispersing.

Remember, building distress tolerance is a vital component of emotional resilience and mental health. By equipping children with playful tools and strategies for coping with difficult emotions, you empower them to navigate life's challenges with greater ease and confidence. So have fun, get creative, and embrace the power of play to transform stress and struggle into growth and joy!

Part 5: Behavioral Modification Play Interventions

CHAPTER 17: HARNESSING THE POWER OF POSITIVE REINFORCEMENT IN PLAY

CHOOSING EFFECTIVE REWARDS AND PRAISE FOR YOUR CHILD

Imagine you're training a baby elephant to lift its foot on command. Would you scold it every time it fails to comply, or would you reward it with treats and cheers when it takes a step in the right direction? Just like our gentle giant friends, children learn best when their efforts are met with positive reinforcement - the strategic use of rewards and praise to encourage desired behaviors.

The logic is simple: actions that are followed by pleasant consequences are more likely to be repeated in the future. By selectively reinforcing your child's positive choices with things they value, you increase the odds that they'll keep up the good work. And by highlighting their specific strengths and successes with authentic praise, you help them internalize a sense of competence and intrinsic motivation.

But not all rewards are created equal. To be effective, a reinforcer must be:

1. Meaningful: The reward should be something your child genuinely desires and looks forward to, not just what you think they should want.
2. Customized: What motivates one child might leave another shrugging. Take time to observe your child's unique interests, preferences, and love languages.
3. Contingent: The reward should be clearly linked to the desired behavior and given only when that behavior occurs. Avoid accidental reinforcement of whining or nagging.
4. Well-timed: Aim to deliver rewards as soon as possible after the positive action, especially for younger kids. The longer the delay, the weaker the association.
5. Novel: Mix up your rewards and keep them special. If screen time becomes an expectation rather than an earned privilege, it loses its motivating power.

What might this look like in practice? Here are some examples of customized, creative reinforcers:

- For the Lego lover: A small mystery kit for each day they complete their chores without reminders
- For the aspiring artist: A fancy new sketchbook and marker set for consistently kind sibling interactions
- For the soccer fanatic: A special one-on-one practice session with Dad for each week of homework completed on time
- For the social butterfly: A sleepover party with friends after a month of improved cooperation with bedtime routines
- For the animal enthusiast: A behind-the-scenes zoo tour for progress made in managing big emotions

The key is to think beyond generic prizes and tie rewards to your child's unique motivations. Involve them in brainstorming ideas and agreeing on clear, achievable behavior targets. The more ownership they feel in the process, the more invested they'll be in following through.

Alongside concrete rewards, targeted praise is a powerful form of positive reinforcement that costs nothing but thoughtfulness. When you notice your child making an effort or handling a challenge well, take a moment to call it out with specific, authentic appreciation:

- "I saw how you took some deep breaths and used your words when your sister annoyed you. That took a lot of self-control!"
- "You worked so hard on that science project, even when it got frustrating. Your persistence really paid off!"
- "I noticed how you invited the new kid to join your game at recess. That was a really kind and welcoming thing to do."
- "Thank you for putting your dishes in the sink without being asked. It shows a lot of responsibility and helps our whole family."

By highlighting the character strengths and values beneath your child's actions, you help them build a positive self-concept grounded in their efforts and choices. You show them that their contributions matter and that you notice the little things they do to make the world a bit brighter.

Just be sure to keep your praise focused on the process rather than the person. Instead of a generic "You're so smart," try "I can see how much thought you put into that story - the characters really came to life!" This growth-oriented feedback emphasizes skills and strategies that are within your child's control rather than inborn traits or outcomes.

With a treasure trove of meaningful rewards and a commitment to catching your child being good, you're well on your way to becoming a positive reinforcement pro. In the next section, we'll explore how to integrate these powerful tools into your play routines for maximum fun and impact. By rewarding good behavior, you'll help your child develop intrinsic motivation and self-discipline that will serve them long after the sticker charts are retired.

PLAYFUL WAYS TO DELIVER POSITIVE REINFORCEMENT

Now that you've grasped the basic principles of positive reinforcement, it's time to get creative with your delivery! Weaving rewards and praise into your child's natural play environment can make the learning process feel less like a chore and more like an exciting game. By tapping into their imaginative spirit and sense of adventure, you'll keep them engaged and motivated to keep up the good work.

Here are some playful ideas for integrating positive reinforcement into your daily routines:

1. Sticker Charts with a Twist

Instead of a generic grid, create a themed sticker chart that aligns with your child's interests. For the aspiring astronaut, map out a journey to the moon, with each milestone representing a new phase of the mission. For the bookworm, design a reading passport where each sticker moves them closer to a literary destination. Let them choose the stickers and help decorate the chart for added investment.

2. Caught Being Good Jar

Introduce a special jar or box where you can leave little notes catching your child demonstrating target behaviors. Use colorful paper and stickers to make it visually appealing. At the end of each day or week, please read the notes aloud and celebrate their successes together. For older kids, please encourage them to add their self-praise notes when they notice themselves making good choices.

3. Magic Wand of Reinforcement

Create a special "magic wand" (or sword, fairy godmother, or any other theme) that grants bonus points or privileges when your child exhibits positive behaviors. Whenever you catch them being helpful, kind, or responsible, give the wand a theatrical wave and announce the reward with flair: "By the power of the Cooperation Wand, I, at this moment, grant you an extra 15 minutes of playtime!" Make it a fun, impromptu part of your interactions.

4. Strength Scavenger Hunt

Please make a list of your child's positive character traits and hide clues around the house that lead them to discover each one. At each stop, please leave a little note with specific examples of how they've demonstrated that strength. For example, "Clue #1: You showed great patience when you helped your little brother tie his shoes, even though it took a long time." The final clue can lead to a special prize or activity that celebrates their efforts.

5. Cooperative Reward Adventures

Create a shared goal or challenge that the whole family works towards, with a fun group reward at the end. For example, set a target for a certain number of acts of kindness or chores completed, and track your progress together on a big poster. When you reach the goal, celebrate with a special outing or experience that everyone enjoys, like a picnic in the park or a backyard obstacle course.

6. Praise Charades

Turn your positive feedback into a playful guessing game. Give specific praise for good behavior, but instead of naming the child, act it out in charades-style gestures. "I noticed someone being very RESPONSIBLE this morning by packing their backpack without being reminded. Can you guess who it was?" This adds an element of fun and gets everyone looking for the good in each other.

7. Victory Dances and High-Fives

Create a special victory dance, handshake, or cheer that you do together whenever your child makes a good choice or overcomes a challenge. It could be a silly hop, a funky hand jive, or a personalized chant. The physical act of celebrating together reinforces the positive feelings and makes it a more memorable experience.

Remember, the goal is not to turn every interaction into a performance or constantly shower your child with prizes. Aim for a balance of planned and spontaneous reinforcement, and make sure your praise is always grounded in authentic observation and appreciation. And don't forget to model gracious compliment-receiving yourself—it's an important skill for kids to learn!

Most importantly, keep it light and playful. If your reward systems start to feel like a burden or a bribe, take a step back and reevaluate. The best reinforcement arises naturally from a loving, respectful relationship and a shared sense of fun.

With a little creativity and a lot of heart, you can make positive reinforcement a joyful, integral part of your family culture. By consistently noticing and celebrating your child's good choices, you'll help them develop a strong inner compass and a lifelong love of learning. And who knows - you might find yourself doing a little victory dance of your own along the way!

EXERCISE 1: STICKER CHART CLIMBING WALL

Objective:

This activity motivates children to work towards a larger goal by earning small rewards for incremental progress and positive behaviors.

Materials:

- Large poster board or paper
- Markers or crayons
- Stickers
- Tape or adhesive putty

Instructions:

1. Introduce the concept of a sticker chart as a way to track progress and celebrate successes on the way to a big goal. Discuss how small steps can add up to major accomplishments over time.

2. Work with the child to identify a specific, measurable goal they want to achieve, such as completing a certain number of homework assignments, achieving a new skill, or displaying positive behavior consistently.

3. On the large poster board or paper, draw a climbing wall or mountain with a clear starting point at the bottom and the goal at the top. Divide the wall into incremental steps or challenges to be completed along the way.

4. Label each step with a mini-goal or behavior that will earn a sticker, such as:

- Complete one homework assignment
- Practice the new skill for 15 minutes
- Use a calm voice instead of yelling
- Help a family member with a chore
- Go to bed on time without a reminder

5. Choose a theme for the stickers that match the child's interests, such as favorite animals, characters, or symbols. Let the child help select or decorate the stickers to increase their investment.

6. Display the sticker chart climbing wall in a prominent location, such as on the fridge or in the child's room. Provide a container of stickers nearby for easy access.

7. Each time the child completes a step or displays the target behavior, celebrate their progress and let them place a sticker on the corresponding space. Use behavior-specific praise to reinforce their efforts, such as "Great job focusing on your homework and finishing it on time!"

8. As the child nears the top of the climbing wall, build anticipation and excitement for reaching the ultimate goal. Discuss how good it feels to persist and achieve something challenging.

9. When the child reaches the top, celebrate their success with a special reward or privilege that was agreed upon in advance. Take a photo of the completed chart and display it as a reminder of their accomplishment.

Tips:

- Break larger goals into small, achievable steps to maintain motivation and prevent discouragement. Aim for a balance of challenge and success.
- Use a variety of stickers or rewards to keep the chart engaging over time. Consider adding bonus challenges or surprises along the way.
- Involve the child in tracking their progress and placing the stickers to build a sense of ownership and autonomy. Avoid using the chart as a threat or punishment.
- Adapt the chart format to the child's developmental level and interests. Younger children may do better with a simple, linear chart, while older children may respond to a more complex game board design.

EXERCISE 2: COOPERATION CASH

Objective:

This activity reinforces prosocial behaviors and teamwork skills by providing immediate, tangible rewards during cooperative games and activities.

Materials:

- Craft materials for making play money (paper, markers, stickers, etc.)
- Small prizes or privileges to be purchased with the play money
- A variety of cooperative games or activities

Instructions:

1. Introduce the concept of Cooperation Cash as a way to recognize and reward positive social behaviors during group play. Discuss the importance of teamwork, communication, and fairness in cooperative games.

2. Work with the child or group to create a set of play money using paper bills or coins decorated with stickers, drawings, or stamps. Decide on a name and denominations for the currency, such as "Kindness Coins" or "Friendship Bucks."

3. Brainstorm a list of prosocial behaviors or teamwork skills that will earn Cooperation Cash during games, such as:

- Sharing materials or taking turns
- Offering encouragement or praise to others
- Helping a struggling teammate
- Compromising or finding a win-win solution
- Using a calm voice and kind words
- Following the rules and being a good sport

4. Choose a variety of cooperative games or activities that require collaboration and communication, such as team puzzles, group art projects, or partner obstacle courses.

5. Before each game or activity, review the target behaviors and the amount of Cooperation Cash that can be earned for displaying them. Provide each child with a small wallet or envelope to collect their earnings.

6. During the game or activity, provide behavior-specific praise and immediate rewards of Cooperation Cash for any instances of the target skills. Be sure to catch each child displaying positive behaviors and distribute the cash evenly.

7. At the end of the game or activity, have children count and compare their Cooperation Cash earnings. Encourage them to reflect on what they did well and what they could improve next time.

8. Allow children to save and spend their Cooperation Cash on small prizes or privileges, such as a special snack, extra screen time, or a coveted toy. Determine the "prices" in advance and display them clearly.

9. Keep track of the group's cumulative Cooperation Cash earnings over time and set a larger goal to work towards, such as a class party or field trip. Celebrate milestones along the way and discuss how small acts of cooperation add up.

Tips:

- Use Cooperation Cash to reinforce positive behaviors during daily activities and routines, not just during structured games. Look for opportunities to catch children being good throughout the day.
- Provide behavior-specific praise along with cash rewards to help children connect their actions to the outcomes. Avoid using cash as a bribe or a substitute for genuine appreciation.
- Ensure that the prizes or privileges are appealing and motivating for the children but not so valuable that they lead to competition or hoarding. Emphasize the social rewards of cooperation over the material ones.
- Adapt the Cooperation Cash system to different settings and age groups by adjusting the target behaviors, currency values, and reward options. Get creative with the theme and design to match children's interests.

EXERCISE 3: GUESS THE GOOD DEED

Objective:

This activity promotes perspective-taking and empathy by having children identify and appreciate prosocial behaviors in others through a fun guessing game.

Materials:

- Index cards or slips of paper
- Pens or pencils
- A container or envelope for collecting the cards

Instructions:

1. Introduce the concept of a good deed as an action that benefits others or makes the world a better place.

Discuss why it's important to notice and appreciate when others do kind things, even if they don't seek recognition.

2. Give each child several index cards or slips of paper and a writing utensil. Ask them to think of a time when they noticed someone else (a family member, friend, teacher, or stranger) doing a good deed, either for them or for another person.

3. Have the children write down the good deed on a card without naming the person who did it. Encourage them to provide enough detail so that others can guess what happened, but not so much that it gives away the identity. For example:

- "This person helped a classmate who was being bullied."
- "This person donated food to a family in need."
- "This person spent time with an elderly neighbor who was lonely."

4. Collect the completed cards in a container or envelope, shuffling them to mix up the entries.

5. Have children take turns drawing a card from the container and reading the good deed aloud to the group. The other children try to guess who might have done the deed based on what they know about that person's character and past actions.

6. After several guesses, have the child who wrote the card reveal the answer and provide any additional context or details. Encourage the group to express appreciation and admiration for the person's kindness and generosity.

7. Continue playing until all the cards have been read and discussed. Reflect on any common themes or patterns in the good deeds that were shared.

8. Challenge the children to go out and perform their good deeds in the coming week, either for someone they know or for a stranger. Have them write down their experiences to share at the next game session.

9. Over time, keep track of the cumulative good deeds performed by the group and celebrate milestones or remarkable acts of kindness. Discuss how small, everyday actions can ripple out to create a more compassionate world.

Tips:

- Model the activity by sharing your examples of good deeds you've witnessed or performed. Be specific and heartfelt in your appreciation to set the tone.
- Encourage children to look for good deeds in unlikely places or from unexpected sources, such as a younger sibling, a grumpy neighbor, or a busy cashier. Help them see the humanity in everyone.
- Use the game as a springboard for discussions about empathy, compassion, and social responsibility. Explore how it feels to be on the giving and receiving end of a good deed.
- Adapt the activity for different age groups or settings by adjusting the complexity of the deeds or the guessing format. For younger children, you may need to provide more prompts and support in identifying and describing good deeds.

EXERCISE 4: MAGIC MULTIPLIER

Objective:

This activity incentivizes positive behaviors and effort by providing variable reinforcement during games and activities.

Materials:

- A game or activity that involves spinning a spinner or rolling a dice
- A set of behavior goals or effort metrics
- Stickers, tokens, or other small rewards

Instructions:

1. Introduce the concept of the Magic Multiplier as a special power that can increase the value of a player's turn or effort in a game based on their positive behaviors or attitude.

2. Choose a game or activity that involves an element of chance, such as spinning a spinner or rolling a dice to determine the number of spaces to move or points to earn.

3. Create a list of specific, observable behaviors or effort metrics that will trigger the Magic Multiplier during the game. For example:

- Encouraging or complimenting another player
- Persisting through a challenging task or setback
- Following the rules and being a good sport
- Putting in extra effort or creativity
- Displaying a positive attitude or growth mindset

4. Assign a multiplier value to each target behavior based on its difficulty or importance. For example, a simple behavior like following directions might earn a 2x multiplier, while a more challenging behavior like resolving a conflict peacefully might earn a 5x multiplier.

5. During the game or activity, have an adult or designated "spotter" watch for instances of the target behaviors or efforts. When a player displays one of these behaviors, announce that they have activated the Magic Multiplier for their next turn.

6. On the player's next turn, have them spin the spinner or roll the dice as usual. Then, multiply the resulting number by the Magic Multiplier value earned earlier. For example, if the player spun a 3 and earned a 2x multiplier for encouraging another player, they would move 6 spaces instead of 3.

7. Provide immediate, behavior-specific praise along with the multiplied reward to help the player connect their actions to the outcome. For example, "Because you showed great sportsmanship by congratulating your opponent, you get to multiply your next spin by 2! Way to be a good friend."

8. Keep track of the number of Magic Multipliers earned by each player throughout the game or activity. Celebrate players who earn the most multipliers or who display exceptional positive behaviors.

9. After the game or activity, debrief with the players about their experiences with the Magic Multiplier. What did it feel like to be rewarded for their efforts and attitudes, not just their luck or skills? How might they apply this mindset to other areas of their life?

Tips:

- Use the Magic Multiplier sparingly and unpredictably to maintain its novelty and impact. Avoid overusing it to the point where it loses its "magic."
- Tailor the target behaviors and multiplier values to the specific needs and goals of your players. Focus on behaviors that are challenging but achievable for each individual.
- Involve players in creating the list of target behaviors and multiplier values to increase their buy-in and motivation. Allow them to suggest new behaviors or adjust the values over time.
- Apply the Magic Multiplier concept to other types of reinforcement beyond game points, such as earning extra privileges, tokens, or stickers for positive behaviors throughout the day.

Remember, positive reinforcement is most effective when it is immediate, specific, and meaningful to the individual child. By incorporating playful, variable rewards into everyday activities and interactions, you can help children develop intrinsic motivation and a growth mindset that will serve them well beyond the game board. So have fun, be creative, and watch the magic of positive reinforcement unfold!

CHAPTER 18: SETTING CONSISTENT LIMITS AND CONSEQUENCES THROUGH PLAY

ESTABLISHING CLEAR RULES AND EXPECTATIONS

Picture this: You're playing a board game with friends, but nobody bothered to read the rules first. Players are making up their steps, arguing over every turn, and accusing each other of cheating. The game quickly devolves into chaos and hurt feelings, and everyone leaves frustrated and confused. It's not exactly a recipe for a fun game night.

Now, imagine your child navigating playtime without clear guidelines or expectations. They're left to guess what's acceptable and what crosses the line, testing limits to see what they can get away with. When misbehavior inevitably arises, you find yourself reacting inconsistently - sometimes ignoring it, lashing out in anger, sometimes giving in to keep the peace. It's a recipe for power struggles, resentment, and insecurity on both sides.

Just like any good game, playtime thrives on clear, consistent rules that everyone understands and agrees to uphold. When children know what's expected of them and what happens when they veer off track, they feel safer and more secure. Limits provide a predictable structure that frees them up to be creative, take healthy risks, and internalize self-discipline over time.

So, how can you establish clear rules and expectations during playtime? Here are some tips:

1. ***Keep it simple.***
Aim for no more than 3-5 key rules that apply across all play situations. Too many rules can overwhelm kids and set them up for failure. Focus on broad guidelines that cover the most essential bases, like respecting people and property, using kind words, and taking turns.

2. ***State rules positively.***
Frame your expectations in terms of what you want to see rather than just what you don't want. Instead of "No hitting," try "We use gentle touches." Instead of "Don't be rude," try "We use friendly words." Positive phrasing gives kids a clear target to aim for and reinforces good behavior.

3. ***Make rules specific and observable.***
Avoid vague or subjective language that leaves room for interpretation. "Be good" or "Don't be annoying" mean different things to different people. Clarify specific actions you expect, like "Use an indoor voice" or "Keep your hands to yourself." If you can see or hear it, it's easier to enforce consistently.

4. ***Involve your child in rule-setting.***
Engage your child in a conversation about why rules are important and what expectations they think are fair. Ask for their input on specific guidelines and listen to their perspective. When kids have a say in creating the rules, they're more likely to buy in and take ownership of following them.

5. ***Post rules visually.***
Please write down your agreed-upon rules and post them in a visible spot, like on the fridge or a playroom wall.

Use simple language and pair each rule with a visual icon for pre-readers. Having a concrete reference point makes it easier to refer back to the rules calmly and consistently when reminders are needed.

6. Model rule-following through play.

Show, don't just tell! Demonstrate respect, kindness, and turn-taking in your play behavior. When you make a mistake (because we all do), own it and model making amends. "Oops, I interrupted you - that wasn't respectful. Let me try again and listen to your whole idea." Kids learn more from what we do than what we say.

7. Reinforce rules proactively.

Don't just wait for misbehavior to mention the rules. Point out instances of good rule-following and show appreciation. "I noticed how you shared the blue marker with your sister - that was kind and fair!" Positive reinforcement makes it more likely kids will repeat those behaviors in the future.

Despite your best efforts at prevention, there will still be times when your child tests the limits or outright defies the rules. That's when clear, logical consequences become your best friend. In the next section, we'll explore how to choose and implement consequences that are proportionate, respectful, and directly related to the misbehavior.

Remember, the goal of limits and consequences is not to punish or control but to teach and guide. By approaching discipline with empathy, firmness, and a focus on problem-solving, you help your child develop the self-regulation skills they need to thrive in the world. By grounding your rules in a foundation of love and respect, you create a haven where your child can learn and grow through both their successes and their mistakes.

FOLLOWING THROUGH WITH LOGICAL CONSEQUENCES

Alright, so you've established clear, positive rules for playtime and modeled them consistently. But then, in a moment of frustration or impulsivity, your child chucks a toy at their sibling's head or scribbles all over the walls in permanent marker. Now what? Do you lecture them sternly, send them to their room indefinitely, or throw up your hands and let them slide?

The truth is, no matter how clearly you communicate your expectations, kids will still test the limits and make poor choices sometimes. They're impulsive, egocentric creatures still learning to regulate their big feelings and desires. When misbehavior happens, it's an opportunity to teach them that their actions have consequences - both for themselves and others.

But not all consequences are created equal. Punishments that are arbitrary, harsh, or unrelated to the offense (like getting grounded for a week for not sharing a toy) tend to breed resentment and rebellion rather than real learning. Kids may comply out of fear at the moment, but they're not internalizing self-discipline or empathy.

Logical consequences, on the other hand, are directly connected to the misbehavior and aim to repair the harm done or teach a specific skill. They're proportionate to the offense, respectful in delivery, and give kids a chance to take responsibility for their actions. Some examples:

- If a child throws a toy in anger, they must take a break from that toy until they can use it safely. "I can't let you play with the blocks right now because you threw them. You can try again when you feel calm and ready to build kindly."
- If a child makes a mess on purpose, they must clean it up before moving on to another activity. "You dumped out all the puzzle pieces, and now they're scattered everywhere. Please put them back in the box so we can find them next time we want to play."
- If a child refuses to share a game with their sibling, they must choose another solo activity for a while. "It looks like you're not ready to take turns with the cards right now. Why don't you play with your action figures until you feel more cooperative?"

Notice how each consequence is framed as a result of the child's choice, not an arbitrary punishment imposed by the parent. There's no shaming or blaming, just a calm, matter-of-fact statement of what needs to happen to make things right. The focus is on repairing damage, restoring safety, and practicing positive skills, not on making the child feel bad about themselves.

Of course, delivering consequences consistently in the heat of the moment is easier said than done. It's tempting to react with anger, lectures, or empty threats when your child pushes your buttons. However, responding with harshness or inconsistency only escalates power struggles and erodes trust. Kids need to know that you can handle their biggest feelings and mistakes with composure and care.

Here are some tips for following through with logical consequences respectfully:

1. Take a deep breath.

Pause and regulate your own emotions before responding to misbehavior. It's okay to take a minute to collect yourself or even walk away briefly if you're about to lose your cool. Model self-calming so your child can learn to do the same.

2. Reconnect before correcting.

Suppose your child is dysregulated or defiant; first, aim to restore a sense of safety and connection. Validate their feelings, offer a hug, or sit with them calmly until the storm passes. Only when they feel understood and supported will they be open to learning from the situation.

3. Clarify the rule and reason.

Calmly restate the rule that was broken and why it's important. Keep it short and specific, focusing on the behavior rather than the character. "We agreed not to splash water out of the tub because it makes the floor slippery and unsafe. I know you were having fun, but we need to keep our play safe for everyone."

4. State the consequence clearly.

Explain the logical result of their actions in a neutral, factual tone. Avoid lengthy lectures, sarcasm, or "I told you so"s. "Now we need to pause our bath play so we can clean up the puddles together. You can try again tomorrow to keep the water in the tub where it belongs."

5. Follow through calmly.

Once you've stated a consequence, stick to it with quiet confidence, even if your child protests or bargains. Repeat your expectations like a broken record, empathizing with their disappointment but holding the line. "I know it's frustrating to stop playing, but the rule is we clean up our messes before moving on. I'll be here to help when you're ready."

6. Offer a redo.

Whenever possible, give your child a chance to try again and practice positive behavior. This reinforces that mistakes are opportunities for learning and growth, not permanent failures. "Now that we've cleaned up the water, would you like to show me how you can scoop and pour gently into the tub? I bet you've got some great ideas for keeping it contained!"

Remember, logical consequences are not a magic wand that will eliminate all misbehavior overnight. Like any new skill, self-discipline takes time, practice, and patience to develop. There will be setbacks and relapses along the way, and that's okay. What matters is the overall climate of consistency, respect, and trust you create through your approach to discipline.

By grounding your consequences in empathy and focusing on solutions, you teach your child that their choices matter and that they have the power to make things right. You show them that your love and acceptance are unconditional, even when their behavior is not. And you model the kind of respectful problem-solving and accountability that will serve them well in all their relationships.

So the next time your little one tests a limit or makes a mistake during play, take a deep breath and see it as an opportunity for growth - both theirs and yours. With consistency, compassion, and a commitment to logical consequences, you'll help them develop the inner compass they need to navigate life's challenges with integrity and resilience. You might also find yourself growing in patience and perspective along the way.

EXERCISE 1: HOUSE RULE HOPSCOTCH

Objective:

This activity reinforces important house rules and expectations through a fun, active game that children can play indoors or outdoors.

Materials:

- Sidewalk chalk or masking tape
- List of house rules or behavior expectations
- Small stone or beanbag for tossing

Instructions:

1. Introduce the concept of house rules as guidelines that help everyone in the family feel safe, respected, and responsible. Discuss why consistent rules and consequences are important for creating a positive home environment.

2. Work with your child to generate a list of 5-10 key house rules or behavior expectations, such as:

- Use kind words and indoor voices
- Clean up after yourself
- Ask permission before using someone else's belongings
- Do your chores and homework before screen time
- Tell the truth and take responsibility for your actions

3. Using sidewalk chalk or masking tape, create a hopscotch board on the floor or ground, with one house rule written in each square. Make the squares large enough to accommodate the length of the rule and the size of the child's feet.

4. Explain the rules of House Rule Hopscotch: the child will toss a small stone or beanbag onto the first square, then hop through the board, avoiding the square with the marker. When they reach the end, they will turn around and hop back, pausing to pick up the marker on the way.

5. As the child hops through the squares, have them read each house rule aloud. If they struggle with a word or concept, provide support and clarification as needed.

6. If the child completes the hopscotch board without touching any lines or losing their balance, they earn a small reward or privilege, such as a sticker or an extra minute of playtime.

7. Play multiple rounds of House Rule Hopscotch, with the child tossing the marker onto different squares each time. Encourage them to see how many rounds they can complete without mistakes.

8. After the game, debrief with the child about the house rules they reviewed. Ask them to reflect on why each rule is important and how following the rules helps the family function better.

9. Display the list of house rules in a visible location, such as on the fridge or in the child's bedroom, as a reminder of the expectations. Refer back to the House Rule Hopscotch game as a fun way to review and reinforce the rules regularly.

Tips:

- Adapt the house rules and consequences to your family's specific needs and values. Use positive, age-appropriate language that focuses on what to do rather than what not to do.
- Allow your child to help create the hopscotch board and decorate it with colorful drawings or stickers related to each rule. This can increase their ownership and engagement with the activity.
- Use the hopscotch game as a regular check-in or reminder system, such as playing it once a week or whenever a rule is repeatedly forgotten or challenged.
- Extend the activity by having your child create their hopscotch boards with rules for other settings, such as the classroom, playground, or community. Discuss how different contexts may have different expectations, but the underlying principles of respect and responsibility are constant.

EXERCISE 2: IF-THEN SPINNER

Objective:

This activity teaches children about the logical consequences of their choices and actions through a fun, unpredictable game.

Materials:

- Paper plate or cardboard circle
- Markers or crayons
- Scissors
- Brad fastener or pencil to create a spinner
- List of "If" scenarios and corresponding "Then" Consequences

Instructions:

1. Introduce the concept of consequences as the natural or logical results of our choices and actions. Discuss how every decision we make has a consequence, whether positive or negative.

2. Work with your child to brainstorm a list of common "If" scenarios that they might encounter, such as:

- If you complete your chores on time...
- If you hit your sibling...
- If you tell the truth about a mistake...
- If you forget to brush your teeth...
- If you share your toys with a friend...

3. For each "If" scenario, generate a corresponding "Then" consequence that logically follows from the action. Focus on natural, reasonable consequences rather than arbitrary punishments. For example:

- If you complete your chores on time, then you can have extra screen time.
- If you hit your sibling, then you must apologize and do something kind for them.
- If you tell the truth about a mistake, then we can work together to fix it.
- If you forget to brush your teeth, then you must do it before bedtime story.
- If you share your toys with a friend, then you can choose the next game to play.

4. Create an If-Then Spinner by dividing a paper plate or cardboard circle into wedges and writing an "If" scenario in each section. Attach a spinner arrow in the center using a Brad fastener or pencil.

5. Play the If-Then Spinner game by having your child spin the arrow and read aloud the "If" scenario it lands on. Then, work together to decide on the logical "Then" consequence that follows.

6. Discuss how the consequence fits the action and why it is important. Help your child understand the reasoning behind the consequences and how it can help them make better choices in the future.

7. Take turns spinning the arrow and generating "Then" consequences for each "If" scenario. Encourage your child to think creatively and realistically about the outcomes of different choices.

8. After playing the game, display the If-Then Spinner in a visible location as a reminder of the connection between actions and consequences. Refer back to it when discussing real-life situations and decisions.

Tips:

- Use the If-Then Spinner to prompt discussions about hypothetical scenarios and decision-making skills. Encourage your child to think through the potential consequences of their choices before acting.
- Create multiple spinners for different contexts or themes, such as school, friendships, or health. This can help your child understand how consequences apply across different areas of life.
- Involve your child in generating the "If" scenarios and "Then" consequences to increase their ownership and understanding of the concept. Allow them to add new scenarios or modify the spinner over time.
- Use the spinner as a positive reinforcement tool by including more scenarios with desirable outcomes, such as "If you help your sibling with their homework, then you can choose the movie for family night." This can motivate your child to make responsible choices proactively.

EXERCISE 3: CONSEQUENCE CARDS

Objective:

This activity reinforces the connection between actions and consequences in a playful, imaginative way that encourages children to think before acting.

Materials:

- Index cards or cardstock
- Markers or pens
- Decorative materials (stickers, washi tape, etc.)
- Container or envelope for storing cards

Instructions:

1. Introduce the concept of Consequence Cards as a fun way to explore what might happen if we make certain choices or display certain behaviors. Emphasize that the consequences in the game are pretended and exaggerated, but they can still teach us important lessons about real life.

2. Work with your child to generate a list of silly or imaginative consequences for various actions, both positive and negative. For example:

- If you share your lunch with a friend, you will sprout wings and fly!
- If you tell a lie, your nose will grow longer like Pinocchio's!
- If you clean your room without being asked, a magical fairy will leave a surprise under your pillow!
- If you forget to say "please" and "thank you," you will turn into a frog until you learn manners!
- If you help someone in need, you will be granted three wishes by a genie!

3. Write each consequence on a separate index card or piece of cardstock, along with a simple illustration or decoration. Make the cards colorful, fun, and age-appropriate for your child.

4. Place the completed Consequence Cards in a container or envelope, and invite your child to draw one card at

random.

5. Read the card aloud and act out the consequence together, using props, costumes, or silly voices as desired. Encourage your child to be creative and imaginative in their portrayal of the consequences.

6. After acting out the consequence, discuss the underlying message or lesson it teaches about real-life behaviors and choices. Help your child connect the silly consequence to a more realistic outcome or rule.

7. Take turns drawing and acting out Consequence Cards, with each person adding their flair and interpretation to the scenarios.

8. Over time, add new cards to the deck based on your child's interests, experiences, or behavior challenges. Use the cards as a lighthearted way to reinforce important lessons and expectations.

Tips:

- Balance the positive and negative consequences in the deck to avoid a punitive or discouraging tone. Focus on the benefits of good choices as much as the drawbacks of poor ones.
- Use the Consequence Cards as a storytelling prompt, encouraging your child to invent a narrative around the character and situation depicted on the card. This can help them develop empathy and perspective-taking skills.
- Adapt the consequences to your child's developmental level and sense of humor. Younger children may enjoy more fantastical or slapstick consequences, while older children may appreciate subtler or more ironic scenarios.
- Create a special ritual or game around the Consequence Cards, such as drawing one card at bedtime or using them as a silly icebreaker at family gatherings. Keep the tone light and playful, even when addressing serious topics.

Remember, the goal of setting limits and consequences through play is to help children internalize positive behavior patterns and develop self-discipline in a way that feels engaging and meaningful to them. By using games, humor, and creativity to explore the ideas of actions and reactions, you can make the learning process more memorable and enjoyable for everyone involved. So have fun, be silly, and watch your child's understanding of consequences grow through the power of play!

CHAPTER 19: TEACHING NEW SKILLS ONE PLAYFUL STEP AT A TIME

BREAKING DOWN COMPLEX SKILLS INTO MANAGEABLE STEPS

Think back to the last time you learned a complex new skill, like playing an instrument, speaking a foreign language, or driving a car. Did you dive in and expect to master it all at once? Of course not! You likely started with the basics, practiced each component separately, and gradually put the pieces together into a fluid whole. Learning any intricate behavior requires breaking it down into digestible chunks and tackling them one at a time.

The same principle applies when teaching your child social-emotional skills through play. While it's tempting to jump straight to the end goal ("I just want them to share nicely!"), expecting perfection right off the bat is a recipe for frustration on both sides. Instead, try using a task analysis approach to dissect the desired behavior into its parts and shape them incrementally.

Let's take the example of turn-taking during a board game. A task analysis might break this skill down into the following steps:

1. Set up the game and choose a player to go first.
2. Roll the dice or spin the spinner when it's your turn.
3. Move your piece to the correct number of spaces.
4. Follow any instructions or actions required by the space you landed on.
5. Pass the dice or spinner to the next player clockwise.
6. Wait patiently and watch attentively while other players take their turns.
7. Respond appropriately when others land on special spaces (e.g., cheer, groan).
8. Keep taking turns until the game is over, following the rules throughout.
9. Congratulate the winner and thank the other players for the game.
10. Help clean up the game pieces and put them away.

Whew, that's a lot of steps for something we often take for granted! However, for a child who struggles with impulse control, cooperative play, or social norms, each of these components may need to be explicitly taught and rehearsed. By focusing on one step at a time and reinforcing successive approximations, you build momentum and set them up for success.

Here's how you might use playful prompts and modeling to shape turn-taking behavior:

1. Start with a simple, fast-paced game that naturally reinforces turn structure, like Go Fish or Snap. The model politely asked for cards and passed them back and forth.

2. Use visual cues like a "my turn" card or token to concretely represent when it's each player's turn. Point to the card and enthusiastically announce "My turn!" or "Your turn!" as you play.

3. When your child gets distracted or interrupts during your turn, gently redirect them: "It's still my turn, but yours is coming up next! Can you watch closely and see what card I draw?"

4. If they try to grab the dice or spinner out of turn, playfully block them and remind them of the rules: "Oops, we have to wait until Mommy's turn is all done before we spin again. Let's sing the 'wait my turn' song while we wait!"

5. Exaggerate your reactions when they successfully wait for their turn: "Wow, you watched so patiently while I moved my piece! That was awesome turn-taking. High five!"

6. Gradually fade your prompts and cues as they get the hang of the routine, but continue to praise their efforts: "I noticed you passed the dice right to your sister when your turn was over without any reminders! You're really getting good at this."

The key is to stay one step ahead of your child's current mastery level, stretching them just enough to keep them engaged but not overwhelmed. If they seem bored or restless with a skill, try upping the challenge by moving to a more complex game or adding silly variations. If they're consistently struggling or melting down, dial it back to a simpler version or take a break and try again later.

It may feel painstakingly slow to teach skills in such small increments, but the payoff is worth it. By breaking complex behaviors into bite-sized pieces and practicing them repeatedly in a playful context, you're laying a strong foundation for generalization and independence. Over time, all those little successes will snowball into a big leap in their social-emotional competence.

So the next time you're tempted to lecture or despair when your child botches a skill, take a deep breath and get curious instead. What tiny step could you zoom in on and reinforce right now? How could you make practicing that step so irresistibly fun that they can't help but try again? With a little creativity and a lot of compassionate persistence, you'll be amazed at how quickly those building blocks stack up into impressive new abilities.

CHAINING STEPS TOGETHER THROUGH ENGAGING GAMES AND ACTIVITIES

Alright, so you've got the hang of breaking skills down into parts and reinforcing baby steps - go, you! But what about stringing all those steps together into a smooth sequence? How do you help your child internalize the flow of a complex behavior until it becomes second nature?

Enter chaining: the process of linking discrete actions into an integrated whole through strategic practice and reinforcement. Just like a physical chain is made up of many small links, a behavioral chain connects individual steps into a fluid routine. And what better way to forge those links than through purposeful play?

The key to successful chaining is to start small and gradually build complexity, always keeping the end goal in mind. Break the skill into chunks that make sense functionally, and practice putting them together in a variety of engaging ways. The more your child rehearses the sequence in different playful contexts, the stronger those neural pathways will become.

Let's return to our turn-taking example. Once your child has mastered the basic steps of rolling the dice, moving their piece, and passing to the next player, you can start chaining those actions together into longer sequences. *Here are some playful ways to practice:*

1. Create a silly obstacle course that mimics the flow of a board game. Set up "spaces" with hula hoops or pillows, and use a giant cardboard die or spinner. Players have to perform a funny action at each space before moving on (e.g., hop on one foot, make a silly face). Coach your child to complete their action, then pass the die and cheer on the next player.

2. Play "Board Game Charades." Write down common game actions on slips of paper (e.g., rolling the dice, moving ahead two spaces, drawing a card). Take turns acting out the steps in order, exaggerating the motions and facial expressions. See how many steps you can string together before breaking character!

3. Make up a "Turn-Taking Rap." Compose a silly rhyme that outlines the steps of good turn-taking, set to a catchy beat. Chant it together as you play, pointing to each player as their turn comes up. "Roll the dice, move your man, pass it on as fast as you can! Watch and wait, no debate, till your turn comes back around, mate!"

4. Design a "Good Sport" board game together. Brainstorm common scenarios that arise during games (e.g., landing on a penalty space, getting close to winning) and decide how a good sport would respond. Create cards with these scenarios and place them around a homemade game board. As players land on each space, they have to act out the good sportsmanship skill before moving on.

The beauty of chaining is that it naturally reinforces each step as part of a larger sequence. By practicing the skills in a meaningful order and providing plenty of enthusiastic feedback, you help your child experience the intrinsic rewards of smooth, successful turn-taking. They start to anticipate what comes next and derive pleasure from nailing the flow.

As your child gets more comfortable with the basic sequence, you can up the ante by introducing variations and challenges. Maybe you play a game with more complex rules, like Monopoly Junior, or join a playdate with peers who have different turn-taking styles. Please encourage your child to apply their skills flexibly and problem-solve when hiccups arise.

Remember, the goal is not robotic perfection but fluid adaptability. Expect setbacks and missteps along the way, especially when the context shifts. But with each playful repetition, your child is internalizing the underlying structure and logic of turn-taking, not just memorizing a rigid script.

So keep getting creative with those chaining games! Invent wacky races where players have to collaborate and take turns to reach a shared goal. Host a "Game Show Night" where contestants win points for demonstrating specific sportsmanship skills. The more you can harness your child's natural interests and sense of humor, the more motivated they'll be to keep practicing.

With patience, persistence, and plenty of playfulness, you'll gradually see your child's choppy turn-taking transform into a smooth, sophisticated dance. They'll start initiating the steps on their own, generalizing the skills to new settings, and even coaching others on the finer points of fair play. Best of all, they'll come to associate cooperative gameplay with joy, connection, and a deep sense of mastery.

So here's to the power of chaining through play—may it link your child's learning into a strong, shining bond of social-emotional awesomeness! May it remind us all that even the most complex skills are really just a series of tiny triumphs strung together with love and laughter. Happy gaming!

EXERCISE 1: BALLOON BREATHING

Objective:

This activity teaches children deep breathing techniques for relaxation and self-regulation through a playful, embodied exercise.

Materials:

- Space to move around freely
- Optional: Real or imaginary balloons

Instructions:

1. Introduce the concept of balloon breathing as a way to calm our bodies and minds when we feel stressed, anxious, or overwhelmed. Discuss how deep breathing can help us slow down, focus, and regulate our emotions.

2. Ask your child to stand up tall with their feet shoulder-width apart and their arms relaxed at their sides. Encourage them to imagine they are a balloon, ready to be filled with air.

3. Guide your child to inhale slowly and deeply through their nose, as if they are filling their balloon body with air. As they inhale, have them raise their arms gradually overhead, mimicking the expansion of a balloon.

4. Encourage your child to hold their breath and their balloon arms for a count of three, feeling the fullness and stillness in their body.

5. Guide your child to exhale slowly and completely through their mouth, as if they are releasing the air from their balloon body. As they exhale, have them lower their arms back down to their sides, mimicking the deflation of a balloon.

6. Repeat the balloon breathing cycle several times, emphasizing the slow, smooth, and complete nature of each inhale and exhale. Encourage your child to focus on the sensations of their breath and their body throughout the exercise.

7. After several rounds of balloon breathing, invite your child to check in with their body and mind. How do they feel different from when they started? What do they notice about their breath, their heartbeat, their muscles, or their thoughts?

8. Discuss how balloon breathing can be used as a tool for self-regulation in various situations, such as before a test, during a conflict, or when feeling overwhelmed. Brainstorm specific scenarios where your child can practice using this technique.

Tips:

- Model the balloon breathing exercise alongside your child, exaggerating the movements and sounds to make it more engaging and interactive.
- Use visual aids or props, such as real balloons or pictures of inflating and deflating objects, to help your child connect with the imagery and sensations of the exercise.
- Adapt the pacing and language of the guidance to your child's age and attention span. For younger children, use shorter phrases and more playful cues. For older children, offer more detailed instructions and opportunities for reflection.

- Incorporate balloon breathing into your daily routines, such as during transitions, before bedtime, or as a brain break during homework. The more your child practices this skill, the more easily they will be able to access it when needed.

EXERCISE 2: SKILL SEQUENCE SCRAMBLE

Objective:

This activity breaks down complex skills into smaller, manageable steps and helps children practice sequencing and memory through a hands-on, kinesthetic game.

Materials:

- Index cards or strips of paper
- Writing utensils
- Container or envelope for cards
- Optional: Relevant materials or props for skill demonstration

Instructions:

1. Introduce the concept of skill sequencing as the process of breaking down a complex skill or task into smaller, ordered steps. Discuss how learning new skills can feel overwhelming at first but becomes easier when we take it one step at a time.

2. Choose a specific skill or task that your child is currently learning or struggling with, such as tying shoes, making a sandwich, or solving a math problem. Break this skill down into 5-7 discrete, observable steps.

3. Write each step of the skill on a separate index card or strip of paper, using clear, concise language and numbering the steps in order. For example, the steps for tying shoes might be:

1. Cross laces

2. Tuck one lace under the other

3. Pull tight

4. Make a loop (bunny ear) with one lace

5. Wrap the other lace around the loop

6. Push the second lace through the hole

7. Pull tight and adjust

4. Mix up the step cards and place them in a container or envelope. Explain the Skill Sequence Scramble game to your child: they will draw the cards one at a time, put them in the correct order, and then demonstrate the skill using the sequenced steps.

5. Have your child draw the step cards from the container and lay them out in a line, rearranging them until they are in the proper order. Offer guidance or hints as needed, but encourage your child to use their memory and

logic to figure out the sequence.

6. Once the steps are properly sequenced, have your child read each step aloud and mime or demonstrate the corresponding action. Use relevant materials or props as needed to make the demonstration more concrete and engaging.

7. Repeat the sequence several times, with your child drawing and arranging the cards, reading the steps, and demonstrating the skill. Offer praise and feedback on their sequencing and execution of the skill.

8. As your child becomes more proficient with the skill, increase the challenge by adding more steps, using less explicit language on the cards, or timing their performance. Celebrate their progress and mastery of the skill.

Tips:

- Choose skills that are developmentally appropriate and relevant to your child's current needs and interests. Break down the skill into steps that are specific, observable, and achievable for your child's level.
- Use visual aids or illustrations on the step cards to make them more engaging and memorable for your child. Consider color-coding or numbering the cards to reinforce the sequence.
- Adapt the language and complexity of the steps to your child's age and learning style. For younger children, use simple, concrete words and phrases. For older children, incorporate more technical or abstract language as appropriate.
- Extend the activity by having your child create their Skill Sequence Scramble games for skills they have mastered or want to teach others. Encourage them to break down the skill, write the steps, and demonstrate the sequence to a family member or friend.

EXERCISE 3: OBSTACLE COURSE

Objective:

This activity provides a fun, physical way for children to practice and reinforce new skills through a series of challenges and obstacles.

Materials:

- Space to set up an obstacle course (indoors or outdoors)
- Various materials for creating obstacles and challenges (e.g., pillows, hula hoops, jump ropes, cones, tunnels, balance beams)
- Props or equipment relevant to the skill being practiced
- Optional: Timer, scorecard, or reward system

Instructions:

1. Introduce the concept of an obstacle course as a series of physical challenges that require specific skills and strategies to complete. Discuss how obstacle courses can be a fun and active way to practice new skills and build confidence.

2. Choose a specific skill or set of skills that your child is currently learning or working on, such as balance, coordination, hand-eye coordination, or spatial awareness. Brainstorm a list of obstacles and challenges that

could help them practice and demonstrate these skills.

3. Set up the obstacle course in a safe, open space, using a variety of materials and props to create different stations or challenges. Each obstacle should require your child to use the targeted skill in a specific way. For example:

- Balancing on a wobble board or walking heel-to-toe on a line
- Throwing a ball through a hoop or at a target
- Crawling through a tunnel or under a net
- Jumping over hurdles or skipping with a rope
- Navigating a zigzag pattern or weaving through cones

4. Explain the rules and goals of the obstacle course to your child, demonstrating each challenge and skill as needed. Emphasize the importance of safety, persistence, and self-challenge throughout the course.

5. Have your child complete the obstacle course, offering encouragement and feedback on their performance of each skill. Time their run or keep score based on the number of successful challenges completed, if desired.

6. After the first run, debrief with your child about their experience. What skills did they feel most confident with? Which challenges were the most difficult? What strategies did they use to overcome obstacles?

7. Run the course several more times, encouraging your child to beat their own time or score or to focus on improving specific skills. Offer variations or modifications to the challenges as needed to keep the course engaging and appropriately challenging.

8. Celebrate your child's progress and mastery of the targeted skills, emphasizing the value of effort, practice, and perseverance. Discuss how they can apply these skills and strategies to other areas of their life.

Tips:
- Tailor the obstacle course to your child's age, abilities, and interests. Choose achievable challenges that are slightly outside their comfort zone to encourage growth and self-challenge.
- Use positive reinforcement and specific praise throughout the activity, focusing on your child's effort, improvement, and problem-solving strategies rather than just their speed or success.
- Incorporate multiple senses and learning styles into the obstacle course, such as visual cues, auditory signals, or tactile feedback. This can help your child engage with the skills on multiple levels and retain the learning more effectively.
- Make the obstacle course a social activity by inviting friends or family members to participate, cheer, or compete alongside your child. Encourage teamwork, sportsmanship, and mutual support throughout the activity.

Remember, teaching new skills through play is all about breaking down the learning process into manageable, enjoyable steps that engage your child's natural curiosity, creativity, and sense of fun. By using interactive, multisensory activities like balloon breathing, skill sequence scrambles, and obstacle courses, you can help your child develop a growth mindset, a love of learning, and a resilient approach to challenges. So get creative, get active, and watch your child's skills and confidence soar!

CHAPTER 20: REDUCING PROBLEM BEHAVIORS THROUGH POSITIVE REDIRECTION

RECOGNIZING THE FUNCTION OF YOUR CHILD'S CHALLENGING BEHAVIORS

Picture this: You're sitting down for a peaceful family game night, ready to bond over some friendly competition. But before you can even finish setting up the board, your child starts grabbing pieces out of turn, making silly noises to distract others, and getting up every few seconds to spin around the room. When you try to redirect them, they collapse on the floor in tears, shouting, "This game is stupid anyway!" So much for a relaxing evening of quality time, right?

It's easy to get frustrated or take it personally when a child's misbehavior seems to sabotage a perfectly good playtime. But here's the thing: behind every challenging behavior is an unmet need or underdeveloped skill. Kids don't wake up in the morning plotting ways to push our buttons – they're doing the best they can with the tools they have to get their needs met and communicate their struggles.

That's where functional behavior assessment comes in handy. By playing detective and looking for patterns in when, where, and how misbehavior shows up, we can start to form hypotheses about its purpose or "function." We can then use that insight to proactively meet the underlying need more positively, reducing the child's reliance on problematic strategies.

Some common functions of misbehavior during play might include:

1. Attention-seeking: A child who feels disconnected or unseen may act out to get a reaction from others, even if it's a negative one. They may interrupt, clown around, or deliberately break the rules to pull focus back to themselves.

2. Escape/avoidance: A child who feels overwhelmed, bored, or incompetent may act up to escape an activity that's too challenging or not stimulating enough. They may whine, procrastinate, or pick fights to delay or avoid the task.

3. Access to tangibles: A child who struggles with impulse control or delayed gratification may misbehave to get immediate access to a desired toy, treat, or activity. They may grab, whine, or negotiate incessantly to wear down adult resistance.

4. Sensory stimulation: A child who is over- or under-responsive to sensory input may seek out intense or repetitive movements, sounds, or textures to regulate their internal state. They may jump, spin, crash, or chew in ways that disrupt play or bother others.

Of course, most behaviors serve multiple functions at once, and the same action may meet different needs in different contexts. A child who grabs a toy from their sibling might be seeking both social attention and access to the coveted item. A child who runs around the room during a board game might be trying to both avoid a frustrating turn and get some much-needed physical input.

That's why it's so important to put on our curiosity caps and look beyond the surface of the behavior. Instead of jumping to conclusions or reacting punitively, we can ask ourselves: "What might my child be trying to communicate or achieve right now? What skills or supports might they be lacking to meet that need more appropriately?"

Some clues that can help us crack the code:

- Timing: Does the behavior tend to happen at a certain time of day, during specific activities, or in response to particular triggers?
- Environment: Are there any sensory aspects of the setting (e.g., noise level, visual clutter) that might be contributing to dysregulation?
- Interactions: How do others typically respond to the behavior? Does it result in increased attention, escape from demands, or access to desired items?
- Skills: Does my child have the communication, emotional regulation, problem-solving, or social abilities to meet their needs more adaptively?

By piecing together these puzzle pieces, we can start to form a clearer picture of the "why" behind the behavior. Once we understand the function, we can get creative about filling that need proactively before things escalate into a full-blown meltdown.

For example, if a child is acting silly and disruptive during a game, in order to get more interaction and playful engagement, we might try:

- Inviting them to be our "special assistant" and give them a specific role or job to do as part of the game setup or play
- Creating a silly secret handshake or victory dance to do together at key points in the game, meeting their need for shared laughter and physical connection
- Pausing at regular intervals to check in one-on-one, offer specific praise for positive behaviors, or engage in a bit of roughhousing or chase before returning to the game.

By embedding these moments of positive, need-meeting interaction into the natural flow of the game, we can help the child feel seen, valued, and connected without having to resort to negative attention-seeking. Over time, they learn that they can get their needs met through appropriate channels, and the challenging behaviors start to lose their appeal.

Of course, this proactive approach requires us to be flexible, patient, and creative in the moment. It means learning to see challenging behaviors as communication rather than intentional defiance or manipulation. And it often involves slowing down, tuning in, and finding the playful "yes" behind the automatic "no."

But with practice, this positive redirection becomes second nature. We start to anticipate our children's needs and struggles before they boil over and respond with empathy and skill-building rather than frustration or punishment. We learn to work with rather than against our child's unique wiring, temperament, and developmental stage.

Most importantly, we strengthen the foundation of trust, attunement, and joyful connection that allows our child's best self to blossom. By approaching misbehavior with curiosity and compassion, we send the message that all of our child's needs and feelings are valid, even when their actions need some fine-tuning. We create a safe space for them to practice new skills and learn from their mistakes without fear of rejection or shame.

So the next time your child's behavior throws a wrench in your playful plans, take a deep breath and channel your inner detective. What might they be trying to tell you through their actions? How can you fill that need or build that skill in a way that feels loving, connecting, and even fun? With a little creativity and a lot of heart, you might find a playful path through the storm – and come out the other side with an even stronger bond.

PLAYFULLY REDIRECTING MISBEHAVIOR TOWARDS POSITIVE ALTERNATIVES

Alright, so you've done your detective work and have a hunch about the function of your child's misbehavior. Maybe they're climbing all over the furniture during a game in order to get some intense sensory input and physical release. Or perhaps they're grabbing the dice out of turn to gain a sense of control and competence in a frustrating situation.

Now comes the tricky part – interrupting that problematic behavior at the moment and guiding them towards a more appropriate way to meet that need. And to do that without escalating into a power struggle or meltdown? It can feel like defusing a ticking time bomb while juggling flaming chainsaws!

But fear not, dear parent – this is where playfulness and positive redirection come to the rescue. By approaching the behavior with a spirit of lightness, empathy, and creativity, we can often steer things in a better direction without getting sucked into a cycle of negativity. The key is to validate the underlying need while setting a clear boundary around the specific action.

Here's a handy formula for playful redirection:

1. Connect before you correct. Take a moment to attune to your child's emotional state and show that you understand their perspective, even if you don't agree with their behavior. This might sound like, "I know it's really hard to wait for your turn when you have such an exciting idea to share! That frustration is so big in your body right now."

2. Clarify the boundary with empathy. Gently but firmly state the limit on the specific behavior while acknowledging the underlying desire or struggle. For example, "I can't let you grab the dice from your sister, even though it's really tempting when it feels like forever to wait. Everyone must get a fair turn."

3. Redirect to a positive alternative. Suggest a more appropriate way to meet the need, ideally one that feels playful and engaging to your child. This is where you can get creative and tap into their natural interests and motivations! Some examples:

- For the sensory-seeking climber: "Ooh, I see your body needs to move and groove! How about we have a dance party when it's not your turn to help you stay focused? Show me your silliest moves!"
- For the dice-grabbing control seeker: "I know you really want to be in charge of the game. Would you like to be my special 'dice master' and hand them to each player when it's their turn? You can even make a fancy flourish each time!"
- For the distraction-prone wanderer: "I wonder if we could make a special 'waiting spot' next to the board where you can hang out and doodle while you wait? You could even draw a silly picture for each player as a surprise!"

The idea is to channel the impulse into a safer, more constructive outlet that still meets the core need. By offering a choice between two positive options, we give the child a sense of agency and buy-in rather than just shutting down their behavior.

4. Follow through calmly and consistently. Once you've set the limit and offered an alternative, stick to it with quiet confidence. If the child resists or persists in the negative behavior, calmly repeat the boundary and redirect again. Avoid lecturing, shaming, or getting drawn into arguments –keep steering them back to the positive path like a broken record.

5. Praise progress and effort when your child engages with the alternative or shows even a tiny step in the right direction; pile on the specific, enthusiastic praise! Highlight the positive behavior you want to see more of and link it to their internal qualities and the impact on others. "Wow, I love how you used your 'dice master' skills to make sure everyone got a fair turn! You showed so much patience and generosity—that makes the game more fun for everyone!"

The goal is to make the positive alternative feel more rewarding and connected than the negative behavior so that it becomes the go-to choice over time. By consistently meeting the need constructively, we help the child build new habits and skills that serve them better in the long run.

Of course, this takes practice and patience on our part. There will be times when our playful redirection falls flat or when our frustration gets the better of us. In those moments, it's okay to hit the pause button and regroup. We might say something like, "I'm feeling really frustrated right now, and I need a minute to calm down before I can help solve this problem. Let's take a break and come back when we're both ready to try again."

The key is to model self-regulation and repair rather than perfection. By owning our struggles and apologizing when we miss the mark, we teach our children that mistakes are part of the learning process. We show them that it's okay to have big feelings and that we can always find our way back to connection and problem-solving.

Over time, this playful, proactive approach to misbehavior can work wonders. By meeting our children's needs with empathy and creativity, we help them feel seen, supported, and able to handle life's challenges. We teach them that there are many ways to navigate tricky situations and that we're always in their corner, ready to guide them toward the light.

So the next time your child's behavior threatens to derail your playtime, take a deep breath and put on your playful problem-solving hat. Channel your inner Mary Poppins and find the fun in even the most frustrating moments. With a little bit of laughter and a whole lot of love, you can turn those misbehavior lemons into sweet, skill-building lemonade – and build a stronger bond in the process.

Just remember – you've got this. You are the expert on your child's unique needs and strengths, and you have all the tools you need to navigate this wild, wonderful journey of parenthood. So keep shining that light of playful positivity, and trust that your love and creativity will guide the way.

EXERCISE 1: WHEEL OF CHOICES

Objective:

This activity helps children identify and practice appropriate behavior alternatives to common problem behaviors using a fun, game-like format.

Materials:

- A large piece of cardboard or poster board
- Markers, crayons, or colored pencils
- Ruler and pencil
- Scissors
- Brad fastener or pushpin and pencil
- List of problem behaviors and appropriate alternatives

Instructions:

1. Introduce the concept of positive redirection as a way to replace problem behaviors with more appropriate, prosocial actions. Discuss how having a range of positive choices can help children feel more in control and capable of managing their behavior.

2. Work with your child to generate a list of common problem behaviors they exhibit or struggle with, such as hitting, yelling, grabbing toys, or refusing to share. For each problem behavior, brainstorm 2-3 appropriate alternative behaviors that could meet the same underlying need or desire. For example:

- Instead of hitting when angry, try taking deep breaths or asking for space.
- Instead of yelling to get attention, try using a calm voice or tapping someone's shoulder.
- Instead of grabbing toys from others, try asking politely or offering a trade.
- Instead of refusing to share, try setting a timer or finding a way to play together.

3. Draw a large circle on a piece of cardboard or posterboard, using a ruler and pencil to ensure a neat, even shape. Divide the circle into wedges, with one wedge for each set of problem behavior and alternatives.

4. In each wedge, write the problem behavior in one color and the alternative behaviors in another color. Use clear, concise language and simple pictures or symbols to represent each action. Make the positive alternatives larger and more visually prominent than the problem behavior.

5. Decorate the wheel with bright colors, stickers, or other designs that appeal to your child's interests and age level. Make the wheel as engaging and attractive as possible.

6. Attach an arrow to the center of the wheel using a Brad fastener or pushpin and pencil so that the arrow can spin freely around the wheel.

7. Introduce the Wheel of Choices to your child, explaining how to use it when they feel the urge to engage in a problem behavior. They can spin the arrow and practice the positive alternative behavior that it lands on.

8. Model using the Wheel of Choices by acting out a scenario where you feel frustrated or tempted to misbehave. Spin the arrow, read the alternative behavior, and demonstrate how to use it at the moment.

9. Encourage your child to use the Wheel of Choices regularly, both in calm moments and in the heat of emotion. Offer praise and positive reinforcement when they choose an alternative behavior, and help them reflect on how it felt to make a positive choice.

Tips:

- Keep the Wheel of Choices in a visible, accessible location where your child can easily refer to it when needed. Consider making a portable version that they can carry with them or keep in their backpack.
- Adapt the problem behaviors and choices to your child's specific needs and developmental level. Use language and examples that are relevant and meaningful to their daily life.
- Involve your child in creating the Wheel of Choices as much as possible, from brainstorming the alternatives to decorating the wheel. The more ownership they feel over the tool, the more likely they are to use it.
- Use the Wheel of Choices as a springboard for ongoing conversations about behavior, emotions, and problem-solving. Encourage your child to come up with alternative behaviors or to reflect on how different choices lead to different outcomes.

EXERCISE 2: CALM CORNER CAFÉ

Objective:

This activity creates a designated space for children to practice self-regulation and coping skills when they feel overwhelmed or dysregulated.

Materials:

- Small, cozy space in your home or classroom (e.g., corner, tent, or nook)
- Soft seating (e.g., beanbag chair, cushions, or pillows)
- Soothing sensory items (e.g., fidgets, stress balls, soft fabrics, weighted blanket)
- Calming activities (e.g., coloring books, puzzles, picture books, music player)
- Relaxing décor (e.g., twinkle lights, posters, plants, or photos of nature)
- Optional: Refreshments and snacks for a café vibe

Instructions:

1. Introduce the concept of a Calm Corner Café as a special place to go when your child feels overwhelmed, anxious, angry, or dysregulated. Explain that it's a safe space to take a break, calm their body and mind, and practice coping skills before returning to the situation.

2. Choose a small, quiet area of your home or classroom to designate as the Calm Corner Café. Involve your child in selecting the location and setting it up to ensure it feels inviting and comfortable to them.

3. Decorate the Calm Corner Café with soft, cozy seating and soothing sensory items that promote relaxation and self-regulation. Consider including:

- Beanbag chairs, cushions, or pillows for sitting or lying down
- Fidgets, stress balls, or other tactile objects for sensory input
- Soft fabrics, stuffed animals, or a weighted blanket for comfort and security

- Coloring books, puzzles, or other quiet activities for focus and distraction
- Music player with headphones for calming sounds or white noise
- Twinkle lights, posters, plants, or nature photos for a peaceful ambiance

4. Add a few refreshments or snacks to the Calm Corner Café, such as water bottles, herbal tea, or small, healthy treats. This can help create a positive association with the space and encourage your child to view it as a nurturing, rejuvenating place.

5. Teach your child how to use the Calm Corner Café appropriately, emphasizing that it is not a punishment or time-out but a positive strategy for managing big feelings. Model using the space yourself when you feel stressed or overwhelmed.

6. Establish clear guidelines for when and how to use the Calm Corner Café, such as:

- Recognizing signs of escalating emotions in their body or mind
- Asking permission or notifying an adult before going to the Calm Corner Café
- Setting a time limit for the break (e.g., 5-10 minutes) before returning to the situation
- Cleaning up and resetting the space after each use

7. Encourage your child to use the Calm Corner Café regularly, both proactively and reactively. Help them identify triggers or situations that may benefit from a calming break, and prompt them to use the space when you notice signs of dysregulation.

8. After each use of the Calm Corner Café, debrief with your child about their experience. What strategies did they use to calm down? How do they feel different after the break? What would they do differently next time?

Tips:
- Customize the Calm Corner Café to your child's specific sensory needs and preferences. Some children may prefer dim lighting and soft textures, while others may seek out bright colors and active sensory input.
- Include a visual schedule or choice board in the Calm Corner Café to guide your child through the self-regulation process. This can help them feel more in control and focused during their break.
- Rotate the materials and activities in the Calm Corner Café regularly to keep it fresh and engaging. Involve your child in selecting new items or creating their calming tools.
- Use positive reinforcement to encourage and celebrate your child's use of the Calm Corner Café. Offer specific praise for their self-awareness, coping skills, and ability to return to the situation calmly.

EXERCISE 3: PASS THE PARCEL

Objective:

This activity promotes turn-taking, impulse control, and cooperative play through a classic party game with a positive behavior twist.

Materials:

- Small gift or toy
- Several layers of wrapping paper
- Tape or stickers
- Music player
- Timer
- Optional: Small treats or activity cards for each layer

Instructions:

1. Introduce the concept of Pass the Parcel as a game that requires patience, self-control, and teamwork. Explain that players will take turns unwrapping a gift while music plays and that the game is more about the fun of playing together than about who ends up with the final prize.

2. Wrap a small gift or toy in several layers of wrapping paper, securing each layer with tape or stickers. You can include a small treat, sticker, or activity card between each layer to add suspense and excitement to the game.

3. Gather your child and any other players in a circle, either sitting on the floor or around a table. Place the wrapped parcel in the center of the circle.

4. Explain the rules of the game:

- When the music starts, players will pass the parcel around the circle in one direction.
- When the music stops, the player holding the parcel will unwrap one layer of paper.
- If there is a treat or activity card between the layers, the player can keep or complete it.
- The game continues until the final layer is unwrapped and the gift is revealed.

5. Start the music and have players begin passing the parcel. Use a timer or random intervals to stop the music, ensuring that each player gets a chance to unwrap at least one layer.

6. As players unwrap each layer, encourage them to use positive behavior skills such as:

- Waiting patiently for their turn and resisting the urge to grab or rush
- Using gentle hands and respecting the parcel and other players
- Celebrating each other's success and sharing the excitement
- Following the rules and directions of the game
- Displaying good sportsmanship and a positive attitude, win or lose

7. When the final layer is unwrapped, and the gift is revealed, have players discuss how they will share or distribute the prize fairly. Encourage them to use problem-solving and negotiation skills to reach a solution that

feels good to everyone.

8. After the game, debrief with players about their experience. What positive behavior skills did they use or observe during the game? How did it feel to take turns and work together? What was challenging or exciting about the game?

Tips:

- Adapt the Pass the Parcel game to different ages and group sizes by adjusting the number of layers, the type of gift or treats, and the complexity of the rules. For younger children, use fewer layers and simpler instructions.
- Use the game as an opportunity to practice specific positive behavior skills that your child is working on, such as impulse control, emotional regulation, or social communication. Provide specific praise and feedback when you observe them using these skills.
- Make the game more cooperative by having players work together to unwrap each layer or by including group challenges or activities between layers. This can help build a sense of teamwork and shared purpose.
- Use the Pass the Parcel format to teach academic or cognitive skills as well, such as math facts, sight words, or trivia questions. Include skill-based challenges or review cards between each layer to reinforce learning in a fun, engaging way.

Remember, reducing problem behaviors through positive redirection is all about teaching and reinforcing the skills and strategies that help children meet their needs in appropriate, prosocial ways. By using playful, interactive activities like the Wheel of Choices, Calm Corner Café, and Pass the Parcel, you can help your child develop a repertoire of positive behavior alternatives that are both effective and enjoyable. So get creative, stay patient, and celebrate each step towards more peaceful, cooperative interactions!

Part 6: Strengthening Attachment and Family Dynamics

CHAPTER 21: NURTURING SECURE ATTACHMENT THROUGH CHILD-LED PLAY

FOSTERING TRUST AND SAFETY THROUGH UNCONDITIONAL ACCEPTANCE

Imagine for a moment that you had a magic mirror that could show you the deepest corners of your child's heart - their secret fears, their wildest dreams, their unspoken hurts. Would you approach that sacred space with judgment and attempts to control it or with curiosity and unconditional love?

When we invite our children to take the lead in play, we offer them just such a magic mirror. Through their imaginative choices, they reveal the inner landscape of their minds and hearts—the themes that preoccupy them, the feelings they're struggling to express, and the ways they're trying to make sense of their world. By responding to those vulnerable revelations with openness, empathy, and delight, we send a powerful message of safety and acceptance.

Child-led play is all about creating a judgment-free zone where kids can explore the full spectrum of their being without fear of rejection or correction. It's a space where they can be silly, messy, loud, aggressive, tender, creative, or anything in between - and know that they are loved and valued just the same. This unconditional acceptance is the cornerstone of secure attachment, allowing children to develop a deep sense of inherent worth and trust in their caregivers.

What does this look like in practice? Here are some key principles for fostering emotional safety through non-directive play:

1. *Let your child choose the play theme and direction.* Resist the urge to guide them towards activities you think are "healthy" or "productive." If they want to spin in circles for 20 minutes, so be it! If they want to create an epic battle between dinosaurs and fairies, go with it. Their play is their way of processing and communicating what's important to them.

2. *Embrace the dark and the light.* Don't shy away from playing themes that feel uncomfortable or taboo, like death, violence, or bodily functions. These are natural parts of a child's imaginative world and often serve an important emotional purpose. By accepting all of their play without judgment, you create a safe container for them to explore and express their shadow side.

3. *Reflect, don't direct.* Instead of asking leading questions or making suggestions, please describe what you see and hear in their play with curiosity and acceptance. "The dinosaur is really mad! He's stomping and roaring so loudly." "The fairy looks scared. She's hiding behind the tree and crying." This reflective narration shows your child that you're attuned to their inner world without trying to change it.

4. *Delight in their unique imagination.* Let your face and voice express genuine wonder, interest, and pleasure in your child's creative choices. Laugh at their silly jokes, marvel at their clever solutions, and validate their big feelings. Your authentic engagement is the ultimate reward for their self-expression.

5. Join in as a follower, not a leader. If your child invites you into their play, take on the roles and actions they suggest without trying to steer the plot. Let them be the director and you the willing actor. If they hand you a prop and say, "You be the baby," embrace your inner infant and follow their lead!

6. Trust in their self-discovery. Resist the temptation to turn play into a "teachable moment" or impart your adult wisdom. Kids learn best when they're allowed to explore and experiment on their terms. If they're struggling with a challenge or expressing a tough feeling, validate their experience and offer gentle encouragement. "That puzzle is really tricky! You're working so hard to figure it out."

By committing to these nondirective principles, you create an oasis of emotional safety where your child can bring all of themselves and know that they are cherished, flaws and all. This doesn't mean that you never set limits or teach skills—it simply means that you prioritize connection and acceptance, building a foundation of trust that can weather any storm.

Of course, following a child's lead in play is often easier said than done, especially when their choices push our emotional buttons. Maybe we feel anxious when they want to play out scary scenarios or bored when they get stuck in repetitive loops. In those moments, we must regulate our reactions and resist the urge to take control. We can silently remind ourselves that this is their process, not ours and that our job is to bear witness with loving attunement.

The good news is that the more we practice unconditional acceptance, the more natural it becomes. We start to see the world through our children's eyes, delight in their unique quirks and creations, and trust in their innate drive toward growth and healing. And as they feel that unwavering support and delight, they blossom into their fullest, most vibrant selves.

So the next time your child invites you into their imaginative world, take a deep breath and surrender to their lead. Let them be the captain of their ship, knowing that you're the steady anchor they can always return to. By embracing them just as they are, mess and all, you give them the ultimate gift of secure attachment - a north star that will guide them through life's every adventure.

BALANCING AUTONOMY SUPPORT WITH SENSITIVE ATTUNEMENT

As much as child-led play is about giving kids the freedom to explore on their terms, it's not a completely hands-off approach. Even the most independent-minded child needs the reassuring presence of a caring adult to feel truly safe and supported in their play. The key is to strike a delicate balance between respecting their autonomy and providing sensitive attunement - a dance of "serve and return" that builds trust and resilience.

One of the most important ways to support your child's autonomy during play is to follow their lead in terms of engagement. Some kids love having their parents join in as active play partners, while others prefer to explore independently with the reassurance of a caring adult nearby. The goal is to take your cues from your child, respecting their signals about when to step in and when to hang back.

This might look like:

- Observe quietly from the sidelines as your child immerses themselves in solo play, trusting in their ability to entertain themselves and problem-solve on their own.

- Joining in as a co-player when invited, but allowing your child to direct the themes and actions rather than imposing your agenda.
- Offer comfort or encouragement when your child seeks it out, but resist the urge to jump in prematurely at the first sign of frustration or distress.
- Setting clear, consistent boundaries around safety and respect but keeping limits minimal to allow for maximum exploration and self-expression.

The idea is to create a "circle of security" around your child's play - a safe space where they can venture out and explore the world, knowing that you're always there to welcome them back when they need support or reassurance. This secure base allows them to take healthy risks, test their limits, and develop a sense of mastery and independence.

At the same time, providing sensitive attunement means staying closely tuned in to your child's emotional state and responding with empathy and validation. This is where your reflective narration skills come in handy - by putting words to your child's play experiences and inner world, you show them that you "get it," even if you don't always agree or approve.

For example:

- If your child is gleefully bashing two dolls together, you might say something like, "Wow, those dolls are feeling really wild and crazy right now! They're crashing into each other like mighty warriors!"
- If your child is tenderly rocking a baby doll to sleep, you could reflect, "Aww, you're being so gentle and loving with that baby. It looks like she feels so safe and cozy in your arms."
- If your child is growling and stomping around like an angry lion, you might validate, "That lion is feeling so mad and frustrated! His roar is so big and loud - he's really letting those feelings out!"

The goal of this attuned reflection is not to analyze or interpret your child's play but to mirror back their experience with acceptance and understanding. By giving voice to their inner world, you help them feel seen, heard, and validated - even when their feelings or behaviors are messy or challenging.

Of course, there will be times when your child's play pushes the limits of safety or respect, and that's where your sensitive limit-setting comes in. The key is to intervene in a way that maintains connection and autonomy support, even as you redirect their behavior.

For example, if your child is throwing blocks at the wall, you might say something like, "I can see you're feeling really excited and powerful right now! Your arm is so strong when you throw those blocks. And I need to keep our home safe, so let's find a different way to play that doesn't damage the walls. How about we set up some empty boxes as targets and see how many you can knock down?"

By acknowledging the feeling or impulse behind the behavior ("you're feeling excited and powerful") while still holding the boundary ("I need to keep our home safe"), you help your child feel understood and accepted even as you guide them towards more appropriate choices. This collaborative approach builds their capacity for self-regulation and problem-solving rather than relying on external control.

As you practice this balance of autonomy support and sensitive attunement, you may find yourself marveling at the depth and complexity of your child's play. You may witness them working through tough emotions, testing out new identities, or creating elaborate worlds with their unique logic and rules. Through it all, your job is to be a loving witness and haven - to delight in their discoveries, offer comfort when needed, and trust in their innate wisdom.

Over time, this consistent experience of being seen, accepted, and supported in play lays the foundation for a secure attachment that will serve your child throughout their life. They learn that their feelings and experiences are valid, that challenges can be overcome with creativity and persistence, and that they can always turn to you for understanding and encouragement.

Every child has the birthright to this sense of emotional safety and autonomy, and it starts with the simple, profound act of letting them take the lead in play. So take a deep breath, set aside your adult agenda, and marvel at the magic that unfolds when you trust in your child's unique path. With your loving attunement as their guide, they'll learn to navigate the world with confidence, resilience, and an unshakable sense of their worth.

EXERCISE 1: SERVE AND RETURN

Objective:

This activity fosters attunement and connection by having parents follow and mirror their child's lead in play, creating a reciprocal "dance" of interaction.

Materials:

- Open space for play
- Variety of age-appropriate toys or props
- Curiosity and patience

Instructions:

1. Invite your child to engage in free play with you, emphasizing that they get to be the leader and you will be the follower. Let them choose the activity, toys, or props to play with.

2. As your child begins to play, observe their actions, facial expressions, and vocalizations closely. Notice the small details of how they manipulate objects, move their body, or create stories.

3. After watching for a bit, begin to copy or mirror your child's play actions, as if you are serving the ball back to them in a game of tennis. If they stack a block, you stack a block. If they make a silly face, you make a silly face. If they make a sound effect, you make a similar sound effect.

4. Keep your mirroring actions slightly delayed and not identical so that your child can notice and respond to your imitation. The goal is to create a back-and-forth exchange where you are both attuned and responsive to each other.

5. If your child seems to enjoy or be intrigued by your mirroring, keep following their lead and copying their actions. If they seem disrupted or annoyed, pull back and give them space to play independently for a bit before rejoining.

6. As the play evolves, look for opportunities to expand or build on your child's actions while still following their

lead. If they draw a circle, you might draw a circle and add a smiley face. If they pretend to feed a doll, you might pretend to feed a stuffed animal.

7. Allow your child to respond to your expansions and take the play in new directions. The goal is to co-create a joyful, attuned interaction where both of you feel seen, heard, and delighted.

8. After the play session, reflect on what you noticed about your child's interests, skills, and emotional expressions. Share specific moments of connection or attunement that you experienced together.

Tips:

- Let go of any agenda or expectations for the play session. The goal is to be fully present and responsive to your child, not to teach or direct their play.
- Use nonverbal cues like eye contact, facial expressions, and gestures to communicate your interest and attunement. Mirror their energy level and tone as well as their actions.
- Be patient and allow for pauses, repetitions, and tangents in the play. Resist the urge to fill the silence or rush the action. Trust your child's natural pace and flow.
- If you feel silly or self-conscious mirroring your child's actions, embrace the playfulness and vulnerability. Your child will delight in seeing you enter their world so fully.

EXERCISE 2: PRESENT MOMENT PEEK-A-BOO

Objective:

This activity promotes mindfulness and connection by having parent and child take turns noticing and describing small details of the present moment.

Materials:

- A blanket, scarf, or cloth for hiding
- Quiet, comfortable space

Instructions:

1. Invite your child to play a special version of peek-a-boo with you, where you will take turns focusing on the present moment and sharing what you notice with each other.

2. Find a comfortable spot to sit facing each other, with a blanket or cloth between you. Decide who will be the "hider" first and who will be the "seeker."

3. The hider begins by covering their face with the blanket and taking a few deep breaths, tuning into their senses and the details of the present moment. They might notice the feeling of the blanket on their skin, the sound of birds outside, the smell of dinner cooking, or the thought that pops into their mind.

4. When the hider is ready, they slowly lower the blanket to reveal their face, making eye contact with the seeker. They then share one small detail of what they noticed in the present moment, using specific sensory language.

5. The seeker listens attentively and reflectively, using facial expressions and gestures to show their interest and understanding. They might repeat what the hider shared or ask a follow-up question to learn more.

6. The seeker then takes a turn, being the hider, covering their face with the blanket and tuning into the present moment. They share one detail of what they noticed when they revealed their face.

7. Continue taking turns being the hider and seeker, with each person sharing one present-moment observation at a time. Encourage your child to use all of their senses and to describe their internal experiences as well as external details.

8. After several rounds, reflect on the experience together. What was it like to tune into the present moment so closely? What new things did you notice or appreciate? How did it feel to share your observations?

Tips:

- Model mindful observation by using rich, specific language to describe your present-moment experiences. Avoid general statements like "I feel good" or "I see a tree," and instead say things like "I feel a cool breeze on my cheeks" or "I see a tiny ladybug crawling up a leaf."
- Validate and celebrate your child's observations, even if they seem small or mundane. The goal is to cultivate curiosity and appreciation for the simple wonders of the present moment.
- Adapt the activity to your child's developmental level and attention span. For younger children, keep the rounds short and playful, with lots of exaggerated facial expressions and vocal tones. For older children, you can extend the activity by writing down or drawing your observations together.
- Use the present moment peek-a-boo game as a transitional activity between busy parts of the day, such as after school or before bedtime. It can help both parent and child settle into a state of calm, centered connection.

EXERCISE 3: SECRET MISSION

Objective:

This activity deepens the parent-child bond by having the child create a special, imaginative adventure for the two of them to share.

Materials:

- Paper and pencils/crayons for planning
- Props or costumes for the secret mission (optional)
- Sense of adventure and play

Instructions:

1. Invite your child to imagine that they are a secret agent who has been given a special mission that can only be completed with the help of their most trusted partner (you!). Explain that they will get to plan and lead the mission from start to finish.

2. Provide paper and pencils/crayons for your child to brainstorm ideas and create a plan for the mission. Encourage them to think about the goal of the mission, the steps involved, any obstacles or challenges that might arise, and the special skills or tools that will be needed.

3. Ask open-ended questions to help your child elaborate on their ideas and think through the details of the mission. For example, "What kind of disguise will we need to wear?" or "How will we know when we've

completed the mission?"

4. Once your child has a basic plan, help them gather any props, costumes, or materials needed for the mission. This might include things like spy gadgets, treasure maps, secret codes, or disguise elements.

5. When you're both ready, have your child lead you through the secret mission step-by-step. Follow their instructions and play along with their imaginative scenario, asking questions and offering suggestions as appropriate.

6. As you complete each step of the mission, praise your child's creativity, problem-solving, and leadership skills. Highlight moments of teamwork and connection, such as "I love how we figured out that clue together!" or "It feels so good to have a partner I can trust on this mission."

7. If your child gets stuck or frustrated at any point, gently offer support or guidance while still allowing them to maintain control and ownership of the mission. Remind them that mistakes and setbacks are a normal part of any adventure.

8. When the mission is complete, celebrate your success and reflect on the experience together. What was the most exciting or challenging part of the mission? What did you learn about each other or yourselves? How did it feel to work together so closely?

Tips:

- Be fully present and engaged during the secret mission, letting go of any distractions or agenda. This is a special time for you and your child to connect and enter into an imaginative world together.
- Say "yes, and..." to your child's ideas as much as possible, building on their suggestions and adding your playful twists. This shows them that you value their creativity and are a willing co-conspirator in their adventures.
- Take on a supporting role in the mission, letting your child be the leader and expert. Ask them for guidance and direction, and express admiration for their skills and knowledge.
- Consider making the secret mission a recurring activity, with your child creating new adventures for you to share each week or month. You can build on previous missions or create entirely new scenarios each time.

Remember, nurturing secure attachment through child-led play is all about creating a safe, responsive space for your child to explore, express, and connect with you. By following their lead, reflecting their interests, and delighting in their creativity, you show them that they are seen, heard, and valued for who they are. These playful, attuned interactions lay the foundation for a lifetime of trust, resilience, and joy in your relationship. So have fun, be present, and embrace the magic of child-led play!

CHAPTER 22: DEEPENING EMPATHY THROUGH IMITATION AND REFLECTIVE DIALOGUE

HONORING YOUR CHILD'S EXPERIENCE BY JOINING THEIR PLAY

Imagine you're a traveler in a foreign land, immersed in a culture with customs and traditions that are entirely new to you. You don't speak the language, you don't know the rules, and everything feels a bit overwhelming and confusing. But then, a kind local approaches you with a warm smile and an outstretched hand. They don't try to lecture you or force you to conform to their ways - instead, they invite you to walk alongside them, to observe and participate in their daily rituals at your own pace. Through this gentle, nonjudgmental guidance, you slowly start to feel more at home in this strange new world.

This is the essence of what it means to join your child's play with empathy and attunement. When you immerse yourself in their imaginative world without trying to control or direct it, you send a powerful message of respect and understanding. You communicate that their inner life is valid and valuable, even if it looks different from your own. By following their lead and attuning to their unique perspective, you foster a deep sense of connection and emotional safety.

What does this look like in practice? Here are some tips for sensitively joining your child's play:

1. Observe and listen first. Before jumping in, take a moment to watch and listen to your child's play. Notice the themes, characters, and emotions they're exploring. Please pay attention to their tone of voice, facial expressions, and body language. This careful observation will give you valuable clues about their inner world and how you can best support them.

2. Imitate their actions and energy. One of the easiest ways to join your child's play is to mirror their actions and emotions. If they're bouncing a ball with excitement, pick up a ball and start bouncing it with the same level of energy. If they're gently rocking a baby doll to sleep, find another doll and join in the soothing motions. By synchronizing with their physical and emotional rhythms, you show them that you're attuned to their experience.

3. Adopt a complementary role. Another way to join your child's play is to take on a role that complements their chosen character or activity. If they're playing doctor, offer to be the patient who needs a check-up. If they're building a block tower, ask if you can be the construction worker who helps them lift the heavy blocks. By taking on a supportive role, you become a collaborator in their imaginative world rather than an instructor.

4. Follow their lead. As you join your child's play, resist the urge to hijack the storyline or impose your agenda. Let them be the director, dictating the scenes, characters, and actions. If they hand you a prop and say, "You be the dragon," embrace your scaly new identity without question. If they want to spend 20 minutes building a meticulous block tower only to gleefully knock it down, go with the flow. Trust that their play has its internal logic and purpose, even if it's not immediately clear to you.

5. Embrace the nonsensical. Children's play is often filled with silly, surreal, or even downright bizarre elements - talking animals, magic powers, and absurd plot twists. Rather than trying to make sense of it all or steer it towards more realistic themes, embrace the fancy and imagination. Join in the silliness with your playful contributions, like giving the stuffed bear a goofy accent or suggesting a wacky new superpower for their character. By validating their sense of humor and creativity, you create a joyful, judgment-free space for self-expression.

As you join your child's play with this spirit of openness and attunement, you may be amazed at the insights and emotional connections that emerge. You may notice themes or struggles that your child hasn't been able to express in words, like a recurring motif of rescue and danger or a poignant enactment of a recent loss or transition. By entering their world with empathy and respect, you gain a precious window into their inner landscape - and the opportunity to offer support and understanding in a way that feels safe and organic.

Of course, joining your child's play with sensitivity and attunement is a skill that takes practice and patience. It can feel uncomfortable or even silly at first to fully immerse yourself in their imaginative world, especially if you're used to being the one in charge. You may struggle with the urge to correct their behavior or steer them towards more "productive" activities. But with time and commitment, you'll start to see the magic that happens when you let go of your adult agenda and delight in your child's unique way of being.

One powerful way to deepen this empathic connection is through reflective narration—a running commentary on your child's play that highlights their intentions, feelings, and strengths. In the next section, we'll explore how this simple yet profound technique can help your child feel seen, heard, and validated on the deepest level.

USING REFLECTIVE NARRATION TO VALIDATE YOUR CHILD'S PLAY PROCESS

Picture this: Your child is fully absorbed in an imaginative play scene, acting out a dramatic rescue mission with their favorite stuffed animals. They're making bold proclamations, sound effects, and sweeping gestures as they race around the room, their faces a mix of determination and glee. It's clear that this play is meaningful and engaging to them - but as a parent, it can be hard to know how to respond in a way that feels supportive without disrupting their flow.

Enter reflective narration - a technique that involves providing a running commentary on your child's play, focusing on the process rather than the content. Instead of asking questions, making suggestions, or praising specific outcomes, you describe what you see and hear in the moment, highlighting your child's intentions, emotions, and strengths.

It might sound something like this:

"Wow, those animals are on a big adventure together! I see them climbing over mountains and swimming through deep rivers. It looks like they're determined to get to their destination no matter what."

"The little bunny seems really scared right now - he's shaking and hiding behind the tree. But his friend the bear is right there by his side, giving him a big hug and telling him it's going to be okay."

"You're working so hard on that drawing! I notice how carefully you're choosing each color and adding lots of tiny details. It seems like you have a really clear idea in your mind of how you want it to look."

By reflecting on the process of their play in this way, you communicate that you're paying close attention and valuing their experience without judging or trying to change it. You help them feel seen and understood on a deeper level, even if they can't articulate their thoughts and feelings in words.

Some key principles to keep in mind when using reflective narration:

1. *Focus on the present moment.* Instead of asking about the backstory or what's going to happen next, comment on what you observe in real time. Use present-tense, action-oriented language to describe the characters, movements, and emotions you see unfolding.

2. *Highlight intentions and emotions.* Look beyond the surface actions to the underlying goals and feelings that seem to be driving the play. Are the characters on a quest for treasure or seeking safety and comfort? Do they seem excited, frustrated, or content in their pursuits? By naming these intentions and emotions, you help your child make sense of their inner world.

3. *Avoid excessive questions or praise.* While it's okay to occasionally ask a clarifying question or offer a sincere compliment, try to keep your narration focused on simple observations rather than judgments or demands for explanation. Too many questions can feel intrusive or disruptive to the play flow, while excessive praise can create pressure to perform or please you.

4. *Embrace silence.* You don't need to narrate every single moment—in fact, leaving plenty of space for quiet observation and independent play is crucial. Aim for a balance between reflecting on key moments and allowing your child to fully immerse themselves in their own experience. Trust that even when you're not actively commenting, your presence and attention are deeply felt and appreciated.

5. *Adjust to your child's preferences.* Some children love having a highly engaged play partner who offers frequent reflections, while others prefer more independent exploration with only occasional commentary. Take your cues from your child's responses and body language, and be willing to adjust your approach based on their unique temperament and needs.

As you practice reflective narration, you may be amazed at the depth of connection and understanding that emerges. You may notice your child's face lighting up with joy and recognition when you put words to their unspoken feelings or see them expanding on the themes you've highlighted in their subsequent play. Over time, they may even start to internalize your reflective language, narrating their play with newfound self-awareness and emotional intelligence.

But perhaps most importantly, by consistently validating your child's play process, you send a powerful message that their inner world is worthy of attention and respect, just as it is. You create a safe, accepting space for them to explore the full range of their humanity - the joys and sorrows, the triumphs and struggles, the light and the shadow. And through this radical acceptance, you nurture a secure attachment that will serve as a foundation for their lifelong resilience and self-worth.

So, the next time you find yourself wondering how to support your child's imaginative play, remember the power of reflective narration. Take a deep breath, set aside your adult agenda, and tune in to the magic unfolding before you. Let your words be a mirror that reflects the beauty and meaning of their experience, trusting that your loving presence is the greatest gift of all. And know that with each moment of empathic attunement, you are planting seeds of connection and confidence that will blossom for years to come.

EXERCISE 1: FAVORITE THINGS FINDER

Objective:

This activity builds empathy and understanding by having parents actively search for and engage with objects that represent their child's unique interests, preferences, and experiences.

Materials:

- A collection of your child's favorite toys, objects, or creative works
- Notebook and pen for reflections
- Curiosity and openness

Instructions:

1. Ask your child to gather a collection of their favorite things from around the house or classroom. This might include treasured toys, artwork, photographs, natural objects, or other items that hold special meaning for them.

2. Spread the collection out in a comfortable, quiet space where you and your child can explore the objects together. Take a few moments to look over the items, noticing their colors, textures, shapes, and any other details that stand out.

3. Invite your child to choose one object from the collection to focus on first. Ask them to tell you about what they love about this object, using questions like:

- What makes this one of your favorite things?
- How do you feel when you play with or look at this object?
- What special memories or experiences does this object remind you of?
- What do you imagine or pretend when you use this object?

4. Listen attentively to your child's responses, using facial expressions, body language, and reflective comments to show your interest and understanding. Avoid judging, correcting, or redirecting their sharing.

5. When your child is finished sharing about the first object, choose another one from the collection that sparks your curiosity. Ask your child's permission to explore the object yourself, using your senses and imagination to enter into their experience of it.

6. Share your observations and wonderings about the object, using "I wonder..." statements and sensory details. For example:

- "I wonder what it would feel like to be this soft, cuddly teddy bear in your arms."
- "I'm noticing all the bright, swirly colors in this painting and imagining the excitement you must have felt while creating it."
- "I wonder what adventures this race car has been on with you and what kinds of speeds and tricks it can do."

7. Invite your child to add to or correct your wonderings, deepening your understanding of their perspective and experience. Continue exploring the collection together, taking turns sharing and wondering about the objects.

8. After the activity, take some time to reflect on what you learned about your child's inner world and what it was like to enter into their experience so fully. Write down any new insights or questions in your notebook.

Tips:

- Approach the activity with a spirit of openness, curiosity, and non-judgment. The goal is not to analyze or interpret your child's interests but to understand and appreciate them more deeply.
- If your child seems hesitant or uncomfortable sharing about an object, don't push or pry. Let them guide the level of disclosure and respect their boundaries.
- Consider doing the activity again with objects that represent your childhood interests and experiences. Sharing your treasured items and memories with your child can deepen mutual understanding and empathy.
- Extend the activity by creating a special display or scrapbook of your child's favorite things. Seeing their interests and experiences reflected so tangibly can boost their sense of self-worth and connection with you.

EXERCISE 2: PLAY REPORTER

Objective:

This activity fosters perspective-taking and emotional attunement by having parents "interview" their child about the meaningful moments and themes in their play.

Materials:

- Notebook and pen for play observations and reflections
- Audio recorder or video camera (optional)
- Play props or costumes for the "reporter" role (optional)

Instructions:

1. During your child's next play session, take on the role of a "play reporter" who has been assigned to cover the exciting stories unfolding in their imaginative world. Let your child know that you'll be observing their play and asking questions to learn more about it.

2. As your child plays, jot down objective observations about their actions, facial expressions, tone of voice, and any dialogue between characters. Try to capture the key details of the story or scenario without interpreting or judging.

3. After observing for a while, approach your child and ask if they would be willing to give you an "exclusive interview" about their play. Use an enthusiastic, curious tone and any props or costumes that might make the interview feel more authentic and engaging.

4. During the interview, ask open-ended questions that invite your child to reflect on the meaningful moments and themes in their play, such as:

- "I noticed that the character you were playing seemed really excited when they found the treasure map. Can you tell me more about what that map means to them and where they hope it will lead?"

- "I saw that the two dolls had an argument and then made up with a big hug. What do you think those characters were feeling during that interaction and how did they work through their problem?"
- "I'm curious about the world you created in your block city. What kind of place is it and what do you imagine it would be like to live there?"

5. Listen attentively to your child's responses, using reflective comments and follow-up questions to show your interest and gain a deeper understanding of their perspective. Avoid offering your own interpretations or solutions unless asked.

6. If your child seems comfortable with it, record parts of the interview using an audio recorder or video camera. Let them know that you value their play stories and want to remember the special details they shared.

7. Close the interview by thanking your child for giving you a "behind-the-scenes" look at their play world. Emphasize how much you enjoyed learning about their unique perspectives and experiences.

8. After the activity, take some time to review your notes or recordings from the interview. Reflect on what you learned about your child's inner world, meaningful themes, and imaginative capacities. Consider sharing your reflections with your child and asking for their feedback.

Tips:

- Let your child's interests and comfort level guide the direction and depth of the interview. Some children may be eager to share extensive details about their play, while others may prefer to keep things brief and general.
- Adapt the "reporter" role to your child's developmental level and interests. Younger children may respond best to a silly, exaggerated reporter persona, while older children may appreciate a more serious, respectful approach.
- Use the interview as an opportunity to validate and celebrate your child's creativity, problem-solving, and emotional intelligence. Point out specific moments or themes that impressed you and ask them to elaborate on their process.
- Consider doing a follow-up activity where your child gets to be the "play reporter" and interview you about your own play experiences, either current or from your childhood. Sharing your own play stories can help build a sense of mutual understanding and connection.

EXERCISE 3: WONDER ALOUD

Objective:

This activity models empathy and perspective-taking by having parents verbalize their curious, nonjudgmental observations and questions about their child's play in the moment.

Materials:

- Comfortable, quiet space for play
- Open, curious mindset

Instructions:

1. Join your child in their play space and let them know that you're interested in witnessing and wondering about their play. Emphasize that they are the expert, and you are the learner in this activity.

2. As your child plays, observe their actions, expressions, and dialogue with an open, curious mindset. Pay attention to the small details and unique qualities of their play, as well as any themes or patterns that emerge.

3. Verbalize your observations and wonderings about the play using short, simple statements that begin with "I notice..." or "I wonder..." For example:

- "I notice that you chose the blue block for the top of your tower. I wonder what made you pick that color."
- "I wonder how the puppy feels when the kitten takes his toy away. His face looks sad to me."
- "I notice that you're using a soft, gentle voice for the baby doll. I wonder if she's feeling sleepy or hungry."

4. Aim to make at least one "I notice/I wonder" statement every few minutes, or whenever there is a natural pause in the play. Keep your tone curious and tentative, rather than certain or directive.

5. If your child responds to your wonderings with their own ideas or explanations, listen attentively and reflect back what you hear. Avoid judging or correcting their responses, even if they differ from your own perceptions.

6. If your child does not respond or seems uninterested in your wonderings, simply continue observing and wondering aloud in a gentle, unobtrusive way. Trust that your child is hearing and processing your statements, even if they don't engage directly.

7. Close the activity by sharing a few key things you noticed and wondered about during the play. Emphasize how much you enjoyed getting a glimpse into your child's unique play world and imaginative process.

8. After the activity, take some time to reflect on what you learned about your child's inner experience through your wondering aloud. Consider how you might integrate this curious, nonjudgmental stance into your everyday interactions and observations with your child.

Tips:

- Keep your wondering statements brief and spaced out, rather than peppering your child with constant questions or observations. The goal is to model curiosity and perspective-taking, not to interrogate or interrupt the flow of play.
- Use a warm, gentle tone when wondering aloud, as if you are marveling at a beautiful sunset or interesting cloud formation. This helps create a sense of safety and acceptance for your child to share their inner world.
- If your child corrects or disagrees with one of your observations, thank them for helping you see things from their perspective. This models humility and openness to learning from others.
- Practice wondering aloud during other daily activities beyond play, such as while reading a book together, taking a walk, or trying a new food. This helps generalize the skill of perspective-taking and empathy to multiple contexts.

CHAPTER 23: HEALING DISCONNECTION THROUGH PLAYFUL RECONNECTION

ACKNOWLEDGING RELATIONSHIP RUPTURES WITH HUMILITY AND EMPATHY

No matter how attuned and accepting we strive to be as parents, there will inevitably be moments when we miss our children's cues, misunderstand their needs, or react in ways that leave them feeling hurt, angry, or disconnected. These relational ruptures are a normal and unavoidable part of the parent-child dance - after all, we're only human, and parenting is a messy, imperfect process.

But while ruptures may be inevitable, they don't have to define or damage our relationship in the long run. In fact, when handled with humility, empathy, and a commitment to repair, these moments of disconnection can actually be opportunities to deepen trust and strengthen the attachment bond. By acknowledging our role in the rupture and taking steps to make things right, we teach our children that it's okay to make mistakes, that all feelings are valid, and that healthy relationships can weather conflict and come out stronger.

What does it look like to acknowledge a relationship rupture with humility and empathy? Here are some key principles:

1. Take responsibility for your part. When you realize that you've said or done something that has left your child feeling disconnected or distressed, resist the urge to defend, deny, or deflect. Instead, take a deep breath and own your role in the interaction with a simple, sincere statement like "I messed up" or "I didn't handle that well."

2. Be specific about what you did, not what your child did. Instead of focusing on your child's behavior or reaction, name the specific action or words on your part that contributed to the rupture. For example, "I wasn't listening carefully when you were trying to tell me something important," or "I yelled at you when I was feeling frustrated, and that wasn't okay."

3. Validate your child's feelings. Let your child know that whatever they're feeling in response to the rupture - anger, sadness, confusion, etc. - is valid and understandable. Use reflective language to show that you "get it," even if you don't agree with how they handled those feelings. For example, "I can see why you're so mad at me right now. It doesn't feel good to be ignored or yelled at."

4. Express empathy and remorse. Let your child know that you understand and care about the impact your actions had on them and that you feel sorry for causing them pain. Use "I" statements to take ownership of your own emotions without expecting your child to comfort you. For example, "I feel sad that I hurt your feelings. I never want you to feel like you can't count on me."

5. Commit to making it right. Let your child know that you're committed to repairing the rupture and rebuilding trust, even if you're not sure how to do that yet. Assure them that you'll keep showing up and working to make things better, no matter what. For example, "I know I broke your trust, and I'm going to do my best to earn it back. You deserve a mom who always listens and respects you."

It's important to remember that acknowledging a rupture doesn't mean wallowing in guilt, shame, or self-flagellation. It's not about being a "perfect" parent who never makes mistakes, but rather about being a repairable parent who owns their imperfections with humility and grace. In fact, overcompensating with excessive apologies or dramatic displays of remorse can actually make it harder for your child to authentically express their hurt and anger.

Instead, aim for a tone of calm, respectful ownership that invites dialogue and collaboration. After naming your part in the rupture and validating your child's experience, give them space to share their thoughts and feelings without judgment or defensiveness. Listen carefully and reflect on what you hear, even if it's hard to stomach. Remember that your child is not attacking you as a person but rather expressing their pain and need for reconnection.

If your child is not ready to talk or engage, respect their boundaries and let them know you'll be available when they are. Don't force a premature resolution or demand forgiveness on the spot. Trust that by consistently showing up with empathy and openness, you're laying the groundwork for repairing and rebuilding trust over time.

Of course, acknowledging ruptures is only half the battle - the real healing comes through the concrete actions we take to make things right and re-establish a sense of safety and connection. In the next section, we'll explore some playful strategies for inviting reconnection and rebuilding trust after a rupture through the power of Special Time and lighthearted repair gestures. With a little creativity and a lot of love, we can turn even the most painful disconnections into opportunities for growth and resilience.

INVITING RECONNECTION THROUGH PLAYFUL GESTURES AND SPECIAL TIME

Once you've acknowledged a relationship rupture with humility and empathy, the next step is to actively invite reconnection and rebuilding of trust. And what better way to do that than through the power of play? After all, play is the language of childhood - the realm where hurts can be soothed, bonds can be strengthened, and new possibilities can be imagined.

By infusing our repair efforts with a spirit of playfulness and joy, we create a safe, engaging space for our child to process their feelings and re-establish a sense of closeness and trust. We send the message that even though things got hard, we're still here, we're still delighted by their company, and we're ready to have fun and make new memories together.

One powerful way to invite reconnection through play is to initiate a lighthearted repair gesture that shows your child you're holding them in mind and wanting to make amends. This could be something as simple as drawing a silly picture and leaving it on their pillow or creating a goofy "magic repair wand" that you wave around while chanting a rhyme about your love for them.

The key is to choose a gesture that feels authentic and resonant with your unique child and relationship. Some other ideas:

- Leaving a trail of clues around the house that leads to a cozy "reconciliation fort" stocked with their favorite snacks and activities
- Presenting them with a homemade "coupon book" filled with promises of special one-on-one time, extra privileges, or acts of service

- Performing a silly "apology dance" complete with exaggerated moves and facial expressions
- Writing them a heartfelt letter that owns your mistakes and expresses your unconditional love and commitment to repair

The goal is not to erase the rupture or win your child over with flashy tricks but rather to extend an olive branch and create an opening for reconnection. By approaching the repair process with a sense of playfulness and humility, you disarm defensiveness and create a shared "we're in this together" vibe that can diffuse tension and pave the way for more direct dialogue and problem-solving.

Of course, these one-off repair gestures are no substitute for the ongoing, consistent work of rebuilding trust and connection over time. That's where the practice of Special Time comes in. Special Time is a protected, one-on-one block of time (usually 10-30 minutes) where your child leads the play agenda, and you follow their lead with your full attention and delight. During Special Time, your job is to observe, listen, reflect, and enjoy your child's company without directing the action or trying to teach or correct.

Special Time is a powerful antidote to disconnection because it sends a clear message that your child is worthy of your undivided attention and interest, just as they are. By setting aside your agenda and honoring their unique passions and preferences, you communicate that their inner world matters deeply to you, even when it doesn't match your adult sensibilities. And by delighting in their creativity and agency, you help them feel seen, appreciated, and competent in the driver's seat of their own life.

Some key principles for making Special Time a regular part of your reconnection routine:

1. Make it predictable. Choose a consistent time and place for Special Time each day or week, and protect it fiercely from distractions or interruptions. This predictability helps your child trust that they can count on this special opportunity for connection and self-expression.

2. Let your child lead. Resist the urge to suggest activities or direct the play during Special Time. Instead, let your child choose what they want to do and follow their lead with enthusiasm and openness. If they want to spend the whole time lining up cars or playing the same level of a video game over and over, so be it! The point is to validate their interests and agency.

3. Offer your full attention. During Special Time, put away your phone, forget your to-do list, and bring your full awareness to the moment. Make eye contact, offer reflective observations, and let your face and voice express genuine interest and delight in your child's company. If your mind starts to wander, gently bring it back to the present.

4. Keep it light and playful. Special Time is not the moment for heavy discussions, lectures, or processing of past conflicts. Instead, focus on creating a joyful, connected experience in the here and now. If ruptures or problems do come up, acknowledge them briefly and then redirect the focus back to play: "I know we're still working through that tough moment from earlier. Right now, I want to enjoy being silly together and making some good memories."

5. End on a high note. When the designated time is up, resist the urge to drag things out or slam on the brakes abruptly. Instead, give a gentle 2-minute warning and then wrap up with a special closing ritual like a hug, high-five, or silly dance. Let your child know how much you enjoyed your time together, and affirm your commitment to protecting this special one-on-one time.

By making Special Time a consistent practice, you create an oasis of connection and repair that can help buffer the inevitable ruptures and misattunements of daily life. Over time, your child will come to internalize this experience of being seen, accepted, and celebrated, even in the face of conflict or disconnection. They'll develop a secure sense of attachment that says, "I am loved, I am worthy, and my relationships can withstand the ups and downs of being human."

But perhaps most importantly, Special Time offers you a chance to fall in love with your child anew - to marvel at their quirks, to savor their joy, and to appreciate their unique way of moving through the world. In the midst of the daily grind of chores, homework battles, and sibling squabbles, it can be easy to lose sight of the magic and wonder that drew you to parenting in the first place. By carving out time to delight in your child's essence, you replenish your reserves of patience, perspective, and unconditional love.

So go ahead - break out the silly hats, crank up the tunes, and let your inner child come out to play! With each goofy face and belly laugh, you'll be co-creating a story of resilience and repair that will last a lifetime. And who knows - you might find yourself feeling a little lighter, a little brighter, and a little more connected to your playful spirit in the process.

EXERCISE 1: PEACE OFFERING

Objective:

This activity helps families repair relationship ruptures and rebuild connection after conflicts by extending symbolic gestures of apology, empathy, and goodwill.

Materials:

- Craft materials for making "peace offerings" (e.g. paper, markers, stickers, clay)
- Small tokens or gifts to represent apology and care (e.g. flowers, candy, handmade coupons)
- Open heart and willingness to repair

Instructions:

1. After a conflict or disconnection has occurred in the family, take some time for everyone to cool down and reflect on their role in the situation. Encourage each person to consider how their words or actions may have impacted others and what they could do differently next time.

2. Introduce the idea of making a "peace offering" as a way to extend an olive branch and show the other person that you care about repairing the relationship. Emphasize that a peace offering is not about erasing the hurt or avoiding accountability, but rather about expressing empathy, apology, and willingness to work things out.

3. Invite each family member to create their own unique peace offering using the available craft materials or tokens. Encourage creativity, playfulness, and thoughtfulness in the designs. Some ideas might include:

- A handmade card with a heartfelt message of apology and care
- A coupon book filled with offers of quality time, acts of service, or words of affirmation
- A silly drawing or comic strip that lightens the mood and expresses goodwill
- A small gift or treat that represents the other person's interests or love language

4. When everyone is finished creating their peace offerings, gather together in a calm, neutral space. Take turns expressing any thoughts or feelings about the initial conflict, using "I statements" and reflective listening to ensure mutual understanding.

5. One at a time, have each person extend their peace offering to the other, explaining the meaning and intention behind it. Encourage the receiver to accept the offering with an open heart and express appreciation for the gesture.

6. After all peace offerings have been exchanged, take a few moments to reflect on how it feels to give and receive these tokens of care and repair. What shifted in your bodies, minds, and hearts through this process?

7. Brainstorm any additional steps or agreements needed to fully repair the relationship and prevent similar ruptures in the future. Emphasize the importance of ongoing communication, empathy, and forgiveness in maintaining strong family bonds.

8. Close the activity with a playful, connecting ritual, such as a group hug, high five, or silly dance. Celebrate your family's resilience and commitment to working through tough times together.

Tips:

- Model vulnerability and accountability by being the first to extend a peace offering, even if you were not the primary person at fault in the conflict. This sets a tone of humility and care for others to follow.
- Adapt the peace offering format to your family's unique interests, needs, and love languages. Some families may prefer more verbal or physical expressions of apology, while others may value acts of service or quality time.
- Create a designated space or ritual for exchanging peace offerings, such as a special "reconciliation bench" or "forgiveness fort." This can help make the repair process more concrete and memorable, especially for younger children.
- Practice extending peace offerings for minor ruptures and annoyances, not just major conflicts. This helps build a culture of ongoing repair and connection in the family.

EXERCISE 2: TIME MACHINE

Objective:

This activity helps families practice problem-solving and perspective-taking by imagining alternative ways to handle past conflicts or challenges.

Materials:

- Comfortable, open space for movement and dialogue
- Simple props or costumes to represent different family members or roles (optional)
- Playful, curious attitude

Instructions:

1. Gather the family together and introduce the concept of the "time machine" - an imaginary device that allows you to travel back in time and explore alternative outcomes to past events.

2. Brainstorm a list of recent conflicts, challenges, or disconnections that the family has experienced. Choose one situation to focus on first, making sure everyone feels comfortable and willing to explore it together.

3. Set the scene by briefly recapping what happened in the original situation, including each person's actions, words, and feelings. Keep the tone neutral and objective, avoiding blame or judgment.

4. Imagine that you have now entered the time machine and are traveling back to the moment just before the conflict or challenge arose. Take a few deep breaths and visualize the scene in vivid detail.

5. Invite each family member to take on the role of their past self, using simple props or costumes if desired. Encourage them to embody the thoughts, feelings, and body language of that past self.

6. Begin the scene again, but this time, invite each person to make a different choice or try a new approach to the situation. Encourage creativity, playfulness, and experimentation in the "re-do."

7. Pause the action periodically to reflect on how the new choices are impacting the outcome of the situation. Ask questions like:

- What do you notice about how this choice is making you feel in your body and mind?
- How do you think the other person is experiencing your new approach?
- What ripple effects might this new choice have on the rest of the situation or relationship?

8. Continue playing out the scene, allowing each person to make multiple new choices and experience different outcomes. Encourage a spirit of curiosity and non-judgment as you explore the possibilities.

9. After the scene has reached a natural conclusion, step out of the time machine and debrief the experience together. What insights or "aha moments" did each person have? What new strategies or perspectives might they carry forward into future challenges?

10. Close the activity by affirming each person's willingness to explore alternative perspectives and practice new ways of relating. Celebrate the family's resilience and commitment to growth and connection.

Tips:

- Start with low-stakes, mildly challenging situations and gradually work up to more intense or complex ones as the family builds comfort and skill with the time machine process.
- Encourage each person to focus on changing their own choices and reactions, rather than trying to control or change others. Emphasize personal responsibility and agency.
- If someone gets stuck or frustrated during the re-do, offer gentle coaching or suggestions, but ultimately let them find their own way through the challenge. Trust the process and the wisdom of each person's inner resources.
- Adapt the time machine concept to different learning styles and preferences, such as writing alternative endings to the story, drawing comic strips of new outcomes, or using puppets to represent different perspectives.

EXERCISE 3: HEART LOCK AND KEY

Objective:

This activity helps families express appreciation, affection, and commitment to one another through a symbolic exchange of caring messages and actions.

Materials:

- Construction paper or cardstock
- Markers, stickers, or other decorating materials
- Scissors
- Tape or glue
- Small boxes, envelopes, or containers for the "heart locks"

Instructions:

1. Gather the family together and introduce the concept of the "heart lock and key" - a special way to share heartfelt messages and caring actions with one another.

2. Give each family member a sheet of construction paper or cardstock and invite them to trace and cut out a large heart shape. Encourage them to decorate their heart with colors, pictures, or words that represent their unique personality and love for the family.

3. On the back of the heart, have each person write a special message of appreciation, affection, or commitment to the family. The message could be a favorite memory, a character strength they admire in each person, or a promise for the future. Encourage creativity and heartfelt expression.

4. Next, have each person trace and cut out a small key shape from a contrasting color of paper. On the key, invite them to write down a specific caring action they will do for each family member in the coming week, such as giving a hug, saying "I love you," helping with a chore, or playing a favorite game together.

5. When everyone is finished, have each person fold their heart in half and tape or glue the edges together, creating a "heart lock." They should leave a small opening at the top, just big enough for the key to fit through.

6. Invite each person to take turns delivering their heart lock and key to the other family members, either by placing them in a special mailbox or exchanging them in person. Encourage eye contact, warm touch, and verbal expressions of appreciation during the exchange.

7. After everyone has given and received their heart locks and keys, take a few moments to open the locks and read the messages inside. Share any reactions, reflections, or feelings that arise.

8. Discuss how the family can continue to "unlock" one another's hearts through ongoing expressions of love, gratitude, and kindness. Brainstorm additional caring actions or rituals to try in the future.

9. Display the heart locks and keys in a special place, such as on the fridge or in a family memory book. Let them serve as a visual reminder of the family's unbreakable bond and commitment to nurturing connection.

Tips:

- Adapt the heart lock and key materials to different ages and abilities. Younger children may need help with cutting and writing, while older children and adults may enjoy using more elaborate paper crafting techniques or embellishments.
- Set a regular time, such as weekly or monthly, to repeat the heart lock and key exchange. This helps make expressions of appreciation and affection a consistent part of the family culture.
- Extend the activity by creating heart locks and keys for extended family members, friends, or community helpers. Encourage a spirit of gratitude and kindness that ripples out beyond the immediate family.
- Use the heart lock and key concept to reinforce other family values or practices, such as forgiveness, honesty, or generosity. Create special locks and keys for specific occasions or milestones, such as birthdays, holidays, or achievements.

Remember, healing disconnection through playful reconnection is an ongoing, lifelong process. By incorporating activities like peace offerings, time machines, and heart lock and keys into your family's regular rhythms, you help create a culture of repair, resilience, and unconditional love. These playful practices may feel awkward or silly at first, but over time, they can become powerful tools for navigating the inevitable ups and downs of family life with grace, humor, and compassion. So keep playing, keep connecting, and trust that every small gesture of love and repair is strengthening the bond at the heart of your family.

CHAPTER 24: FOSTERING FAMILY COHESION THROUGH SHARED PLAY RITUALS

ENGAGING THE WHOLE FAMILY IN COOPERATIVE GAMES AND CHALLENGES

In the hustle and bustle of modern family life, it can be all too easy for everyone to scatter to their corners of the house, absorbed in their individual screens, hobbies, or social lives. While each family member needs to have their interests and autonomy, research shows that regular doses of shared fun and togetherness are crucial for fostering a sense of belonging, support, and resilience that can weather life's storms.

One of the most powerful ways to bring the family together and strengthen those bonds is through cooperative play - games and activities that require everyone to work together towards a common goal. Unlike competitive games, where players vie against each other for individual victory, cooperative challenges invite the whole family to pool their unique strengths and ideas in service of shared success.

The benefits of cooperative family play are numerous:

1. Builds teamwork and communication skills. When the family has to collaborate to solve a puzzle, navigate a scavenger hunt, or improvise a skit, they practice vital skills like active listening, clear communication, compromise, and division of labor. These skills translate directly to real-world situations like household chores, sibling conflicts, and major life transitions.

2. Fosters empathy and appreciation for each other. As family members work together and rely on each other's unique contributions, they develop a deeper understanding and respect for each person's perspectives, abilities, and needs. They learn to see each other as valuable allies rather than rivals or burdens.

3. Creates a sense of "we're in this together." Tackling a fun challenge as a united front reinforces the idea that the family has each other's backs, no matter what. It builds a shared identity and sense of camaraderie that can provide a lifelong source of security and strength.

4. Encourages playfulness and laughter. When the family lets loose and gets silly together, it releases endorphins, reduces stress, and creates positive associations with family time. Laughter is a powerful bonding agent that can diffuse tensions, heal rifts, and make even the toughest times feel more bearable.

What does cooperative family play actually look like? Here are some ideas for age-appropriate activities that can get everyone working and laughing together:

- Family Scavenger Hunts: Create a list of clues or challenges that the family has to solve together to find a hidden treasure or reach a final destination. Mix in silly tasks like "take a group selfie with a stranger" or "collect 5 items that start with the letter 'B'" to keep things lighthearted.

- Board Game Tournaments: Choose a series of cooperative board games like Pandemic, Castle Panic, or Hanabi, and play through them as a family, keeping score of your collective successes. Strategize together, cheer each other on, and celebrate your victories with a special treat or dance party.

- Improvised Plays or Music Videos: Give the family a silly prompt or storyline and challenge everyone to come up with characters, costumes, and scenes on the fly. Record your improvised masterpiece and have a family film fest to rewatch your dramatic or musical stylings.
- Cooperative Video Game Nights: Find video games that allow for cooperative multiplayer mode, like Overcooked, Lovers in a Dangerous Spacetime, or Minecraft, and take turns pairing up in teams. Share your favorite strategies and cheer each other through tricky levels.
- Family Service Projects: Look for opportunities to volunteer together at a local food bank, animal shelter, or community cleanup event. Work together to make a difference and reflect on the impact of your shared efforts.

The key to successful cooperative play is to choose activities that are challenging enough to require real collaboration but not so difficult that they lead to frustration or blame. Aim for a mix of silly fun and meaningful purpose, and be sure to celebrate each person's contributions along the way.

As the parent, your role is to be the facilitator and cheerleader of the cooperative spirit. Set the tone by modeling enthusiasm, encouragement, and a focus on process over outcome. If competitiveness or criticism starts to creep in, gently redirect the energy back to the shared goal and the importance of having fun and supporting each other.

With regular practice, cooperative play can become a cherished part of your family culture—a ritual that everyone looks forward to as a source of bonding, laughter, and shared accomplishment. As you strengthen those muscles of teamwork and mutual appreciation, you'll be building a foundation of resilience that will serve your family well through all of life's adventures.

CREATING MEANINGFUL PLAY RITUALS FOR CONNECTION AND CONTINUITY

While one-off cooperative games and challenges can provide a fun boost to family togetherness, there's something uniquely powerful about play rituals woven into the fabric of a family's life. A ritual is more than just a repeated activity—it's an experience imbued with special meaning, anticipation, and a sense of sacred connection. Family play rituals are those cherished traditions that everyone counts on as a source of joy, stability, and shared identity.

Some examples of family play rituals:

- *Friday Night Game Nights*: Every Friday after dinner, the family gathers to play a favorite board game or card game, with silly prizes for the winners and ice cream sundaes for all.
- *Sunday Morning Storytelling:* Every Sunday, over a big breakfast, each family member takes a turn telling a real or imagined story, with bonus points for making everyone laugh or gasp.

- *Full Moon Campfires:* Whenever there's a full moon, the family heads to the backyard or a nearby park for a nighttime campfire, complete with stargazing, silly songs, and s'mores.

- ***Annual Holiday Craft-a-Thons:*** In the weeks before a favorite holiday, the family sets aside time to work on special seasonal crafts together, like carving pumpkins, decorating gingerbread houses, or making Valentine's Day cards.
- ***Monthly "Someday Funday" Adventures:*** On the first Saturday of every month, the family takes turns choosing a special outing or experience to do together, like visiting a new museum, going on a scenic hike, or taking a cooking class.

The beauty of family play rituals is that they provide a reliable source of connection and continuity amidst the ups and downs of life. No matter how hectic the week has been or how much the family has grown and changed, everyone knows they can count on that special time to come together, let loose, and revel in each other's company. It's a way of saying, "This is who we are" and "This is what matters most."

Play rituals can be especially grounding during times of transition or stress, like a move to a new city, a change in family structure, or a global pandemic. When so much feels uncertain or out of control, having those predictable moments of shared joy and silliness can be a lifeline. They remind us that even when the world is turning upside down, we still have each other and the power to create our own pockets of playful magic.

To create meaningful play rituals that stick, consider these tips:

1. Get everyone's input. Bring the whole family together to brainstorm ideas for rituals that everyone would enjoy. What kinds of activities make each person light up? What values or memories do you want to honor? What logistical constraints do you need to work around? The more each person feels ownership over the ritual, the more they'll look forward to and prioritize it.

2. Keep it simple and sustainable. Start with rituals that feel easy and achievable to maintain, like a weekly game night or a monthly movie club. Choose activities that don't require a ton of preparation, supplies, or money, so you're more likely to stick with them even when life gets busy. You can always add more elaborate flourishes over time as the ritual takes root.

3. Protect the time fiercely. Treat your play rituals as non-negotiable commitments, just like school or work obligations. Put them on the calendar, set reminders, and plan around them as much as possible. Of course, there will be times when life intervenes, and you have to skip or reschedule, but aim to make that the rare exception rather than the rule.

4. Add your special touches. Give your play rituals a unique family flair by adding in-jokes, nicknames, silly costumes, or signature snacks. Create funny awards for different categories of contribution, like "Most Creative Cheating" or "Best Evil Cackle." The more personal and quirky the details, the more the ritual will feel like a cherished family heirloom.

5. Evolve with the times. As your family grows and changes, be open to adapting your play rituals to fit new needs and interests. Maybe Friday Night Game Night morphs into Friday Night Karaoke Night when the kids hit their teen years. Maybe Sunday Morning Storytelling can be expanded to include a family podcast. The specific activity matters less than the spirit of playful connection it embodies.

As you weave these play rituals into your family life, you may be amazed at the ripple effects on your overall sense of closeness and well-being. Children thrive on the predictability and specialness of family traditions, and adults often find themselves looking forward to that dedicated playtime just as much as the kids do. Having a consistent source of shared laughter and lightness can make the hard parts of parenting feel more doable, and the sweet parts feel even sweeter.

But perhaps most importantly, by making playful rituals a priority, you're sending a powerful message to your children and yourself about what truly matters in life. In a culture that often worships productivity and individualism over connection and joy, carving out time to delight in each other's company is a radical act of love. It's a way of saying "I choose us" and "I choose to play" over and over again, even in the face of life's demands and distractions.

So go ahead - bust out the silly hats, invent a secret family handshake, and make some magic together. With each goofy giggle and inside joke, you'll be weaving a web of connections that will hold your family together through all of life's twists and turns. And who knows - you might find yourself having so much fun you forget it's good for you.

EXERCISE 1: TEAM HANDSHAKE

Objective:

This activity helps families create a sense of unity, belonging, and team spirit through a special, co-created greeting ritual.

Materials:

- Open space for movement
- Creativity and willingness to be silly

Instructions:

1. Gather the family together and introduce the idea of creating a special "team handshake" - a unique greeting that represents your family's bond and identity.

2. Brainstorm a list of words or values that capture your family's unique qualities, such as love, laughter, adventure, or resilience. Write these down on a large sheet of paper or whiteboard.

3. Next, invite each family member to contribute one or two movements or gestures that could be included in the team handshake. These could be silly, symbolic, or skillful actions, such as high fives, fist bumps, jazz hands, or secret signs.

4. Practice each person's suggested movements one at a time, giving everyone a chance to learn and perfect them. Offer encouraging feedback and celebrate each person's creativity.

5. Once you have a collection of movements, work together to arrange them into a sequence that flows smoothly and feels good to everyone. You may need to try a few different combinations or rhythms before finding the right fit.

6. Add any finishing touches to the team handshake, such as sound effects, chants, or coordinated steps. Make sure everyone has a chance to contribute and feel ownership of the final product.

7. Practice the full team handshake several times until it feels natural and synchronized. Encourage laughter,

playfulness, and a sense of "we're all in this together!"

8. Decide on a name for your team handshake and any special occasions or rituals where you will use it, such as before family game nights, after completing a big project together, or when saying goodbye before school or work.

9. Perform your team handshake with pride and enthusiasm whenever the occasion arises. Let it be a reminder of your family's unique bond and team spirit.

Tips:

- Record a video of your family performing the team handshake so you can watch and enjoy it again later. Share it with extended family or friends to spread joy and a sense of belonging.
- Adapt the team handshake over time as your family grows and changes. Invite new members to contribute their own special moves or modify the sequence to reflect new inside jokes or milestones.
- Use the team handshake as a playful way to reconnect after conflicts or challenges. It can serve as a reminder that, no matter what, you are all on the same team and committed to working through tough times together.
- Extend the team spirit beyond the handshake by creating other family rituals or traditions, such as a special cheer, song, or motto. Wear matching t-shirts or colors to show your family pride and unity.

EXERCISE 2: PROGRESSIVE STORY

Objective:

This activity fosters creativity, collaboration, and a sense of shared family identity through the co-creation of an ongoing, imaginative story.

Materials:

- Notebook or story journal
- Pens or pencils
- Cozy, quiet space for storytelling

Instructions:

1. Gather the family together in a comfortable storytelling spot, such as around the dinner table, on the living room couch, or in a cozy tent or fort.

2. Introduce the idea of creating a "progressive story" together - an imaginative tale that unfolds over time, with each family member taking turns adding to it.

3. Choose a general theme, setting, or genre for the story, such as a fairytale kingdom, a sci-fi adventure, a mystery caper, or a slice-of-life drama. Make sure it's a topic that everyone feels excited and comfortable contributing to.

4. Decide on the opening line or scene of the story, such as "Once upon a time..." or "It was a dark and stormy night..." The first storyteller can elaborate on this opening for a few minutes, setting the stage for the tale to

come.

5. Pass the storytelling baton to the next family member, who picks up where the last one left off and adds their own creative ideas and details to the plot. Encourage each person to build on what came before while also taking the story in new and surprising directions.

6. Continue passing the story around the circle, with each person adding their twist or turn to the unfolding narrative. Set a time limit for each storyteller's turn, such as 3-5 minutes, to keep the pace lively and engaging.

7. As the story progresses, jot down key plot points, character names, or memorable lines in a special story journal. This helps keep track of the evolving narrative and provides a fun record to look back on later.

8. When it's time to wrap up the storytelling session, the last person can leave the tale on a cliffhanger or suggest a satisfying resolution. Decide together whether to continue the same story next time or start a new one.

9. Make the progressive story a regular family ritual, such as a weekly bedtime tradition or a special holiday activity. Over time, you'll build a rich tapestry of shared characters, inside jokes, and imaginative adventures that reflect your family's unique creative spirit.

Tips:

- Encourage each family member to bring their own personality, interests, and experiences to the storytelling process. The goal is not to create a polished, professional tale but to express and celebrate the diversity within your family.
- If someone gets stuck or feels self-conscious about their storytelling skills, offer gentle prompts or suggestions to help them find their flow. Emphasize that there are no "right" or "wrong" contributions, only playful possibilities.
- Consider recording or transcribing the progressive story as an audio or written keepsake. You could even turn it into a homemade book or play, complete with illustrations and character profiles.
- Adapt the progressive story concept to different creative mediums, such as a family comic strip, puppet show, or stop-motion animation. Let your collective imagination run wild!

EXERCISE 3: FAMILY CREST

Objective:

This activity promotes a sense of family identity, values, and pride by inviting members to collaboratively design a symbolic coat of arms.

Materials:

- Large sheet of paper or poster board
- Markers, crayons, or colored pencils
- Magazines, photos, or other collage materials
- Scissors and glue sticks
- Reference images of traditional heraldic symbols

Instructions:

1. Gather the family together and introduce the concept of a coat of arms or family crest - a special shield displaying symbols and colors that represent a family's identity, values, and history.

2. Show some reference images of traditional heraldic symbols, such as lions for courage, eagles for leadership, anchors for stability, or hearts for love. Discuss how these symbols can be combined and arranged to tell a unique family story.

3. Brainstorm a list of values, traits, experiences, and aspirations that define your family. Consider questions like:

- What qualities do we admire and strive for?
- What challenges have we overcome together?
- What are our proudest achievements or fondest memories?
- What dreams or goals do we share for the future?

4. Sketch out a large shield shape on the paper or poster board, leaving space around the edges for additional designs. Divide the shield into four to six sections, either with straight lines or more organic, curving shapes.

5. Invite each family member to choose or create a symbol to represent one of the key family values or experiences brainstormed earlier. Encourage a mix of traditional heraldic images and more personal, creative designs.

6. Draw, paint, or collage the chosen symbols into the different sections of the shield, collaborating to create a balanced, visually striking composition. Add colors, patterns, or embellishments that further express your family's unique style and spirit.

7. Around the border of the shield, add any family mottos, nicknames, inside jokes, or significant dates. These could be written in a fancy script or incorporated into playful, decorative designs.

8. When the family crest is complete, discuss the significance of each element and how it contributes to the overall story and identity of your family. Reflect on what you learned or appreciated about each other through the creative process.

9. Display the finished family crest in a prominent place, such as a living room wall, a scrapbook cover, or a digital screen saver. Let it serve as a daily reminder of your family's shared history, values, and vision.

Tips:

- Make the family crest design an ongoing, evolving project that you revisit and update over time. As your family grows and changes, add new symbols, colors, or elements to reflect your journey.
- Use the family crest as a springboard for other creative projects or adventures, such as a themed family photo shoot, a history or genealogy quest, or a series of "family values" challenges or rewards.
- Create individual "mini-crests" for each family member, showcasing their unique talents, interests, and contributions to the larger family story. Celebrate how each person's quirks and gifts enrich the collective tapestry.

- Extend the family crest concept to other family traditions or milestones, such as a baby naming ceremony, a graduation celebration, or a holiday gathering. Invite extended family or friends to contribute their symbols or stories to the ever-expanding crest.

EXERCISE 4: FLASHLIGHT COMPLIMENTS

Objective:

This activity nurtures a culture of appreciation, affirmation, and emotional safety within the family through a playful, light-hearted ritual.

Materials:

- Flashlight or small lamp
- Comfortable, cozy space with dimmed lighting
- Optional: Soft music or nature sounds

Instructions:

1. Gather the family together in a comfortable, intimate space, such as a living room floor or a backyard tent. Dim the lights or use natural lighting to create a warm, soothing ambiance.

2. Introduce the concept of "flashlight compliments" - a special way of shining a light on the positive qualities and contributions of each family member.

3. Sit in a close circle and pass the flashlight or small lamp to the first family member. Invite them to hold the light and take a few deep breaths, settling into the present moment.

4. Going around the circle, have each family member take turns offering a specific, heartfelt compliment or appreciation to the person holding the flashlight. Encourage a mix of playful, humorous affirmations and more serious, emotional ones.

5. As each person receives their compliments, invite them to soak in the words of affirmation and reflect on how it feels to be seen and celebrated by their family. Encourage them to offer a simple "thank you" or to share any feelings or reflections that arise.

6. After everyone has had a chance to offer their compliments, the person holding the flashlight can share a self-appreciation - something they are proud of or grateful for about themselves. This helps reinforce a sense of intrinsic self-worth and balance the giving and receiving of affirmations.

7. Pass the flashlight to the next family member and repeat the process, ensuring that everyone gets a turn to bask in the warm glow of their family's love and appreciation.

8. Close the activity by reflecting on the power of words to illuminate and uplift each other. Discuss how the family can continue to integrate more authentic, specific compliments and appreciations into their daily interactions.

9. Make the flashlight complement a regular family ritual, such as a weekly check-in or a special holiday tradition. Keep the flashlight or lamp in a central place as a reminder to always be on the lookout for each other's light.

Tips:

- Model vulnerability and emotional safety by going first and offering a heartfelt, specific compliment. Set a tone of authenticity and care that invites others to share from the heart.
- Adapt the ritual to different ages and communication styles by offering sentence starters, visual prompts, or physical gestures to express appreciation. The goal is to make the experience accessible and comfortable for all.
- Record or write down the compliments shared during the ritual to create a beautiful keepsake or reminder of the family's love. Revisit these words of affirmation during tough times or transitions as a source of strength and connection.
- Extend the flashlight compliments to other contexts beyond the family, such as school, work, or community spaces. Encourage family members to be on the lookout for opportunities to shine a light on the goodness in others and themselves.

Remember, fostering family cohesion through shared play rituals is an ongoing, evolving process that requires intentionality, creativity, and a willingness to step outside of comfort zones. By co-creating and regularly practicing rituals like team handshakes, progressive stories, family crests, and flashlight compliments, you weave a rich tapestry of shared meaning, identity, and belonging that can sustain and nourish your family through all the seasons of life. So keep playing, keep connecting, and trust that every small ritual of love and laughter is strengthening the invisible threads that bind you together as a beautifully imperfect, perfectly beautiful family.

CHAPTER 25: PUTTING IT ALL TOGETHER: A FLEXIBLE TOOLKIT FOR PARENTS

MIXING AND MATCHING PLAY THERAPY TECHNIQUES TO FIT YOUR FAMILY

Throughout this book, we've explored a rich tapestry of play therapy approaches and techniques, each offering a unique pathway to healing, growth, and connection. From the child-centered foundations of nondirective play to the structured strategies of cognitive-behavioral interventions, from the mindful presence of attunement to the joyful silliness of family improv games - the possibilities for infusing your parenting with therapeutic play are truly endless.

But here's the beautiful secret: There is no one "right" way to do play therapy at home. Just as every child is unique, every family has its own distinct culture, needs, and strengths that will shape how these ideas come to life in your daily interactions. The most effective and sustainable approach is one that feels authentic and tailored to your specific situation, not one that slavishly follows a pre-set formula from a textbook.

So as you reflect on all the concepts and practices we've covered, I invite you to get curious about what resonates most deeply with your intuition and values. What techniques light you up and make you feel more connected to your child? What philosophies align with your personal parenting goals and beliefs? What activities fit seamlessly into your existing routines and lifestyle?

There is no need to try to implement everything at once or to force yourself to use a strategy that feels contrived or awkward. Trust that you are the expert on your own family and that you have the wisdom and creativity to adapt these ideas in a way that works for you. Give yourself permission to experiment, to mix and match, to put your unique spin on things.

For your family, the core of therapeutic play might look like a daily dose of child-led Special Time, sprinkled with moments of sportscasting and reflective listening. It might also look like a weekly family board game night that integrates cooperative challenges and silly victory dances. It might also look like a monthly "feelings crafternoon" where you break out the art supplies and create characters to represent your inner experiences.

The key is to start small and build on what works, letting your child's engagement and your sense of ease guide you. As you gain confidence and see the positive impact on your relationship, you may find yourself naturally integrating more playful interventions into your everyday interactions.

Here are some prompts to help you create your personalized play therapy toolkit:

1. What are your top 3-5 priorities for your child's social-emotional development right now? (e.g., emotional regulation, problem-solving, self-esteem, cooperation)

2. What play therapy techniques or principles from this book feel most aligned with those goals and your natural parenting style? Make a list.

3. Brainstorm some specific ways you could integrate those techniques into your daily routines and play times in a way that feels fun and manageable. Start with 2-3 simple action steps.

4. Consider your child's unique interests, personality, and developmental stage. What kinds of play activities or themes might they be most drawn to? How could you use those as a starting point for therapeutic interventions?

5. Reflect on your own personal blocks or barriers to engaging in therapeutic play. What mindset shifts or self-care practices could help you show up with more presence and openness?

Remember, the goal is not perfection but progress. Celebrate the small victories, learn from the missteps, and trust that every moment of attuned play is planting a seed for your child's lifelong resilience and well-being.

If you ever feel stuck or discouraged, don't hesitate to reach out for support—whether that's consulting with a play therapist for guidance, swapping ideas with other like-minded parents, or simply taking a deep breath and channeling your inner child. You are not alone on this journey, and there is always room for growth and discovery.

As you continue to explore and customize your family's approach to therapeutic play, I encourage you to embrace a spirit of playful curiosity—both toward your child's inner world and your ongoing development as a parent. In the next section, we'll dive deeper into what it means to bring a beginner's mind and an open heart to this transformative process.

EMBRACING A SPIRIT OF PLAYFUL CURIOSITY AND EXPERIMENTATION

In many ways, embarking on a therapeutic play journey with your child is like setting off on an epic adventure into uncharted territory. You may have a rough map and some helpful tools in your pack, but the real magic happens in the spontaneous discoveries and unexpected detours along the way. Embracing a spirit of playful curiosity means letting go of rigid agendas and being open to the surprises and possibilities that emerge in the moment-to-moment dance of connection.

One of the core principles of play therapy is that children are inherently driven toward healing and growth and that our role as parents and caregivers is to create safe, accepting conditions for that natural wisdom to unfold. But the same is true for ourselves as parents - we each have an innate capacity for learning, evolution, and joyful engagement that is best nurtured through a spirit of open-ended exploration and self-compassion.

Just as we encourage our children to take risks, make mistakes, and try again in their play, we can cultivate that same resilient mindset in our approach to parenting. When we let go of the pressure to "get it right" and instead focus on showing up with authenticity and attunement, we model for our children that growth is a lifelong process, not a fixed destination.

This means permitting ourselves to be beginners, to experiment with different techniques and styles, and to fumble, flop, and giggle our way through awkward moments. It means embracing the messiness and uncertainty of play, trusting that even the "failed" attempts are planting seeds for deeper understanding and connection down the road.

Here are some ways to cultivate a spirit of playful curiosity in your therapeutic play practice:

1. Adopt a beginner's mind. Approach each play session with fresh eyes and an open heart, letting go of preconceived notions or expectations. Be fully present to the unique unfolding of this moment, without comparison to past experiences or future goals.

2. Follow the joy. Notice what activities, ideas, or dynamics light you up and make you feel more alive and connected to your child. Lean into those sparks of delight and let them guide your intuitive, playful choices.

3. Get curious about resistance. When you or your child feel stuck, frustrated, or disconnected, instead of pushing through or giving up, get curious about what's underneath the resistance. What unmet needs, fears, or longings might be driving the behavior? How might you playfully acknowledge and address those underlying factors?

4. Embrace mistakes as learning opportunities. When an intervention flop or an interaction goes awry, resist the urge to blame or shame yourself or your child. Instead, get curious about what you can learn from the experience and how you might approach things differently next time. Model self-compassion and resilience by talking through your thought process out loud.

5. Seek out playful inspiration. Surround yourself with resources, communities, and experiences that fuel your sense of creative joy and wonder. Read books, listen to podcasts, or join groups that celebrate the power of play and offer fresh ideas for engaging with your child. The more you nurture your playful spirit, the more naturally you'll be able to share that energy with your child.

6. Cultivate a gratitude practice. Take time each day to reflect on the small moments of beauty, connection, and growth in your play journey with your child. Celebrate the tiny triumphs, savor the silly smiles, and let those positive experiences fuel your ongoing motivation and commitment.

As you continue to embrace this spirit of playful curiosity, you may find that therapeutic play becomes less of a discrete "technique" and more of an overarching way of being with your child. You may start to see every interaction as an opportunity for connection, every challenge as an invitation for creative problem-solving, and every mistake as a chance for growth and repair.

Along the way, you may discover that this playful approach is not just transforming your child's life but your own as well. By learning to let go of perfectionistic striving and instead lean into the joy and messiness of the moment, you open yourself up to a richer, more authentic way of engaging with the world. You start to see your struggles and setbacks through a lens of compassionate curiosity, and you start to trust in your inherent resilience and capacity for change.

Of course, this process of integration and embodiment is not always a straight or easy path. There will be days when you fall back into old patterns when the demands and stresses of life feel incompatible with a playful mindset, and when you want to throw in the towel and revert to the familiar scripts of control and coercion.

In those moments, remember that even the most experienced play therapists and parents are always learning, growing, and finding their way back to the beginner's mind. The goal is not to be perfect but to be present—to show up for yourself and your child with honesty, humility, and an open heart. Trust that every moment of attuned connection, no matter how small or imperfect, is planting a seed for lifelong resilience and joy.

So, as you close the pages of this book and step into your own unique play therapy journey, know that you are exactly where you need to be. You already have everything you need to create a more playful, connected, and healing relationship with your child. You are part of a larger community of parents and caregivers who are all stumbling, laughing, and learning their way toward a brighter future for our children and ourselves.

CHAPTER 26: CELEBRATING PROGRESS AND MAINTAINING GAINS

TRACKING GROWTH THROUGH REFLECTIVE PLAY OBSERVATIONS

As you and your child embark on your therapeutic play journey, it can be easy to get caught up in the day-to-day challenges and lose sight of the bigger picture. When you're in the trenches of tantrums, power struggles, and emotional upheavals, it's hard to tell if all your playful efforts are actually making a difference. But here's the thing: change is happening, even when it feels imperceptible in the moment. Every small interaction of attunement, every gleeful giggle, every ounce of empathy and understanding you pour into your play is planting a seed for your child's healing and growth.

One of the most powerful ways to stay attuned to this incremental progress is through the practice of reflective play observation. Just as you've learned to observe and reflect on your child's feelings and experiences during a play session, you can bring that same mindful presence to track their growth over time. By intentionally setting aside moments to pause, zoom out, and celebrate the small shifts in your child's play and your relationship, you cultivate a sense of hope, momentum, and long-term perspective.

Here are some prompts to guide your reflective play observations:

1. What new skills or capacities is my child demonstrating in their play?

- Are they showing more imaginative flexibility and coming up with creative solutions to problems?
- Are they expressing their feelings more directly and clearly, using emotional language?
- Are they practicing new coping strategies, like deep breathing or positive self-talk?
- Are they taking more social risks, initiating interactions, or trying out new roles?

2. How have the themes and dynamics of their play shifted over time?

- Are the characters more collaboratively working through challenges rather than fighting or fleeing?
- Are the stories more coherent and organized, with clear goals and resolutions?
- Is there a greater sense of agency and empowerment, with the child taking charge of the narrative?
- Are there more moments of joyful attunement and connection between characters?

3. How have our play interactions felt different lately?

- Do I feel more present, curious, and accepting during our play times?
- Am I less frequently getting stuck in power struggles or negative spirals?
- Are there more moments of shared laughter, silliness, and delight?
- Do I sense a deeper level of trust, openness, and emotional intimacy between us?

4. What new insights or understandings have I gained about my child through our play?

- What unique strengths, interests, and perspectives have I discovered?

- What fears, longings, or unmet needs have I become more attuned to?
- What patterns or triggers have I noticed that help me make sense of their challenging behaviors?
- How has my empathy and appreciation for my child's inner world expanded?

As you reflect on these questions, try to jot down specific examples and anecdotes that illustrate the shifts you're noticing. Maybe you recall a moment when your child spontaneously used a calm-down strategy they learned in play to regulate a big feeling or a story they created about a character persevering through a tough challenge. These concrete snapshots of growth are like little gems you can collect in a journal or scrapbook to revisit and savor over time.

Not only do these reflective observations help you stay attuned to your child's progress, but they also offer a powerful opportunity for celebration and encouragement. By sharing specific examples of growth with your child, you help them build a positive self-narrative and internalize a sense of their resilience and capability. You can say things like:

"Remember when Teddy used his magic breath to calm down when he was feeling frustrated? I saw you do the same thing when your block tower fell yesterday. You're learning so many great ways to handle big feelings!"

"I noticed how the puppets in your story worked together as a team to solve the mystery, even though they had different ideas at first. It reminds me of how well you've been cooperating with your sister lately, even when you disagree. You're really growing in your ability to collaborate and compromise!"

By mirroring back these shining moments and connecting them to their developing skills, you help your child anchor their sense of identity in their strengths and growth rather than their struggles or setbacks. You become their trusted mirror, reflecting the best parts of who they are becoming.

Of course, progress is rarely a straight line, and there will inevitably be times when old patterns resurface, or new challenges arise. In those moments, your reflective observational practice becomes even more crucial as a source of perspective and hope. By widening your lens beyond the immediate hurdle and grounding yourself in the long arc of growth, you can more easily weather the storms and trust in your child's inherent resilience.

It's also important to recognize that your child's progress is inextricably linked to your growth and healing as a parent. By engaging in this reflective practice, you're not just tracking your child's development but also your own expanding capacity for mindful attunement, emotional regulation, and playful connection. You're learning to see yourself through a lens of compassion and curiosity, to celebrate your small victories, and to learn from your missteps.

So, as you continue on this therapeutic play journey, remember to pause often and marvel at the incredible transformations unfolding before your eyes - both in your child and yourself. Trust that every moment of playful presence is weaving a new story of resilience, healing, and connection that will carry you both forward. And know that you are doing the sacred work of nurturing the next generation of compassionate, creative, and emotionally whole humans, one small step at a time.

PLANNING FOR FUTURE CHALLENGES AND CONTINUING THERAPEUTIC PLAY

As you start to see the fruits of your therapeutic play efforts blossoming in your child's increased confidence, resilience, and connection, it can be tempting to sit back and coast on your laurels. When the meltdowns become less frequent, the cooperation becomes more consistent, and the laughter becomes more abundant, it's natural to shift your focus to other pressing priorities and trust that your child has "got it" now. But here's the thing: therapeutic play is not a finish line to be crossed but a lifelong journey of growth and healing. Just as you wouldn't expect to stay physically fit after a few weeks of exercise, your child's emotional muscles need ongoing conditioning and care to withstand life's inevitable challenges.

As your child grows and develops, they will encounter new developmental tasks, social pressures, and environmental stressors that will test their coping skills and sense of self. From navigating the complex social world of school to weathering the hormonal storms of adolescence to launching into the uncharted waters of young adulthood - each stage of life brings its unique challenges that require a foundation of resilience and adaptability. By continuing to prioritize therapeutic play and emotional attunement throughout these transitions, you help your child build an inner reservoir of strength and self-trust that they can draw upon whenever they feel overwhelmed or uncertain.

What does it look like to plan for future challenges and integrate therapeutic play into your long-term parenting approach? Here are some key principles and strategies to keep in mind:

1. Anticipate developmental milestones and transitions. Educate yourself about the typical social-emotional tasks and challenges of each stage of your child's growth, from the separation anxiety of toddlerhood to the identity formation of adolescence. By knowing what to expect, you can proactively adjust your play approach to target the specific skills and capacities your child will need to navigate these transitions smoothly.

2. Adapt play themes and techniques to your child's evolving needs. As your child's cognitive, verbal, and social abilities mature, their play will naturally become more complex and abstract. Follow their lead in exploring new themes, characters, and scenarios that reflect their expanding world and sense of self. Incorporate more sophisticated techniques like role-playing, problem-solving challenges, and symbolic metaphors that align with their developmental level.

3. Gradually fade and scaffold therapeutic supports. As your child internalizes new coping strategies and reaches mastery in certain skill areas, gradually reduce the frequency and intensity of targeted interventions in that domain. Provide just enough support to maintain and generalize gains while giving them opportunities to practice self-sufficiency and self-advocacy. Offer specific praise and encouragement when you notice them applying their skills independently in real-life situations.

4. Prioritize ongoing one-on-one Special Time. Even as your formal play therapy interventions taper off, continue to protect regular blocks of child-led playtime to check in on your child's emotional world and nurture your relationship. These Special Time rituals become even more crucial as your child navigates the increasing complexities of peer relationships, academic pressures, and identity formation. Show up with the same spirit of curiosity, acceptance, and delight, letting your child guide the agenda and pace.

5. Model and practice emotional regulation skills. As your child matures, they will face increasingly sophisticated social and emotional challenges that require a well-honed capacity for self-regulation. Continue to model and practice coping strategies like deep breathing, positive self-talk, and mindfulness in your own life, and invite your child to join you in playful stress-busting activities like yoga, nature walks, or silly dance parties. Normalize talking about big feelings and demonstrate healthy ways of expressing and managing emotions.

6. *Foster open communication and trust.* As your child enters adolescence and beyond, they may naturally start to pull away and seek more independence and privacy. While respecting their need for autonomy, continue to prioritize open, non-judgmental communication and emotional safety. Let them know that you're always available to listen, support, and problem-solve together without trying to fix or control. When conflicts or ruptures arise, lean into your repair skills of empathic listening, humble ownership, and playful reconnection.

7. *Seek additional support when needed.* If your child encounters a particularly challenging situation or developmental hurdle that feels beyond your current capacity, don't hesitate to seek additional support from a play therapist, counselor, or support group. Normalizing the need for extra help models healthy coping and self-care strategies for your child. Collaborating with a trusted professional can give you fresh perspectives, targeted techniques, and a supportive space to process your parenting journey.

Remember, the goal of therapeutic play is not to bubble-wrap your child from all of life's difficulties but to equip them with the inner resources and resilience to weather those challenges with confidence and grace. By continuing to show up for your child with a playful presence, emotional attunement, and an unwavering commitment to growth, you help them internalize a sense of unconditional love and worthiness that will carry them through even the darkest of times.

So, as you look ahead to the winding road of your child's development, trust in the power of play to light the way. Know that every shared giggle, every imaginative adventure, and every tender moment of connection is fortifying your child's roots and expanding their wings. And know that you are not alone on this journey - that there is a whole village of parents, caregivers, and professionals cheering you on and ready to catch you when you stumble.

Most importantly, remember to celebrate the incredible work you are doing each and every day to nurture your child's wholeness and joy. Take time to pause and marvel at the miraculous unfolding of their unique spirit and your blossoming capacity for presence, empathy, and love. Trust that even on the hardest days, you are planting seeds of healing that will bear fruit for generations to come.

So here's to the power of play, the resilience of the human spirit, and the extraordinary love of a parent for their child. May you continue to find joy, wonder, and healing in the sacred space of your shared playfulness today and always. May you always remember that you are enough, just as you are, to give your child the gifts of connection and emotional safety that will carry them through all of life's adventures.

REFERENCE

Burke, C. A. (2010). Mindfulness-based approaches with children and adolescents: A preliminary review of current research in an emergent field. Journal of Child and Family Studies, 19(2), 133-144.

Semple, R. J., Lee, J., Rosa, D., & Miller, L. F. (2010). A randomized trial of mindfulness-based cognitive therapy for children: Promoting mindful attention to enhance social-emotional resiliency in children. Journal of Child and Family Studies, 19(2), 218-229.

Kazdin, A. E. (2001). Behavior Modification in Applied Settings. Waveland Press.

O'Leary, K. D., & Wilson, G. T. (1975). Behavior Therapy: Application and Outcome. Prentice-Hall.

Miller, A. L., Rathus, J. H., & Linehan, M. M. (2007). Dialectical Behavior Therapy with Suicidal Adolescents. Guilford Press.

Fleischhaker, C., Böhme, R., Sixt, B., Brück, C., Schneider, C., & Schulz, E. (2011). Dialectical behavioral therapy for adolescents (DBT-A): A clinical trial for patients with suicidal and self-injurious behavior and borderline symptoms with a one-year follow-up. Child and Adolescent Psychiatry and Mental Health, 5(1), 3.

Kendall, P. C. (1993). Cognitive-behavioral therapies with youth: Guiding theory, current status, and emerging developments. Journal of Consulting and Clinical Psychology, 61(2), 235-247.

Silverman, W. K., & Hinshaw, S. P. (2008). The second special issue on evidence-based psychosocial treatments for children and adolescents: A 10-year update. Journal of Clinical Child & Adolescent Psychology, 37(1), 1-7.

Ray, D. C., Bratton, S. C., Rhine, T., & Jones, L. (2001). The effectiveness of play therapy: Responding to the critics. International Journal of Play Therapy, 10(1), 85-108.

Landreth, G. L. (2012). Play Therapy: The Art of the Relationship. Routledge.

Bratton, S. C., Ray, D., Rhine, T., & Jones, L. (2005). The efficacy of play therapy with children: A meta-analytic review of treatment outcomes. Professional Psychology: Research and Practice, 36(4), 376–390. https://doi.org/10.1037/0735-7028.36.4.376

Cavett, A. M. (2016). Playful Cognitive Behavioral Therapy (CBT). In K. J. O'Connor, C. E. Schaefer, & L. D. Braverman (Eds.), Handbook of play therapy (pp. 315-336). John Wiley & Sons, Inc.

Cornett, N., & Bratton, S. C. (2014). Examining the impact of child parent relationship therapy (CPRT) on family functioning. Journal of Marital and Family Therapy, 40(3), 302-318. https://doi.org/10.1111/jmft.12014

Kestly, T. A. (2016). Presence and play: Why mindfulness matters. International Journal of Play Therapy, 25(1), 14–23. https://doi.org/10.1037/pla0000019

Leblanc, M., & Ritchie, M. (2001). A meta-analysis of play therapy outcomes. Counselling Psychology Quarterly, 14(2), 149–163. https://doi.org/10.1080/09515070110059142

Lin, Y.-W., & Bratton, S. C. (2015). A meta-analytic review of child-centered play therapy approaches. Journal of Counseling & Development, 93(1), 45–58. https://doi.org/10.1002/j.1556-6676.2015.00180.x

Perepletchikova, F., & Goodman, G. (2014). Two approaches to treating preadolescent children with severe emotional and behavioral problems: Dialectical behavior therapy adapted for children and mentalization-based child therapy. Journal of Psychotherapy Integration, 24(4), 298–312. https://doi.org/10.1037/a0038134

Ray, D. C., Armstrong, S. A., Balkin, R. S., & Jayne, K. M. (2015). Child-centered play therapy in the schools: Review and meta-analysis. Psychology in the Schools, 52(2), 107–123. https://doi.org/10.1002/pits.21798

Sanders, M. R., Kirby, J. N., Tellegen, C. L., & Day, J. J. (2014). The Triple P-Positive Parenting Program: A systematic review and meta-analysis of a multi-level system of parenting support. Clinical Psychology Review, 34(4), 337-357. https://doi.org/10.1016/j.cpr.2014.04.003

Swank, J. M., & Smith-Adcock, S. (2018). On-task behavior of children with attention-deficit/hyperactivity disorder: Examining treatment effectiveness of play therapy interventions. International Journal of Play Therapy, 27(4), 187–197. https://doi.org/10.1037/pla0000082

Thomas, R., & Zimmer-Gembeck, M. J. (2007). Behavioral outcomes of Parent-Child Interaction Therapy and Triple P—Positive Parenting Program: A review and meta-analysis. Journal of Abnormal Child Psychology, 35(3), 475-495. https://doi.org/10.1007/s10802-007-9104-9

Zalewski, M., Goodman, S. H., Cole, P. M., & McLaughlin, K. A. (2017). Clinical considerations when treating adults who are parents. Clinical Psychology: Science and Practice, 24(4), 370–388. https://doi.org/10.1111/cpsp.12209

Bowlby, J. (1988). A Secure Base: Parent-Child Attachment and Healthy Human Development. Basic Books.

Hughes, D. A. (2004). Building the Bonds of Attachment: Awakening Love in Deeply Troubled Children. Rowman & Littlefield.

Schaefer, C. E. (2011). Foundations of Play Therapy. Wiley.

VanFleet, R., Sywulak, A. E., & Sniscak, C. C. (2010). Child-Centered Play Therapy. Guilford Press.

* 9 7 8 1 9 6 2 0 2 7 3 3 5 *